Better

Better

How I Let Go of Control,
Held On to Hope, and
Found Joy in My Darkest Hour

Amy Robach

BALLANTINE BOOKS
NEW YORK

Published in the United States by
Ballantine Books, an imprint of Random House,
a division of Penguin Random House LLC, New York.

BALLANTINE and the HOUSE colophon
are registered trademarks of
Penguin Random House LLC.

LIBRARY OF CONGRESS CATALOGING-IN-PUBLICATION DATA
Robach, Amy.
Better : how I let go of control, held on to hope, and found joy in my
darkest hour / Amy Robach.
pages   cm
ISBN 978-0-553-39298-2 (hardback) — ISBN 978-0-553-39299-9 (eBook)
1. Robach, Amy.   2. Television personalities—United States—
Biography.   3. Television news anchors—United States—Biography.
4. Breast—Cancer—Patients—United States—Biography.   I. Title.
PN1992.4.R315A3 2015
791.4502'8092—dc23
[B]
2015025171

Printed in the United States of America on acid-free paper

randomhousebooks.com

2 4 6 8 9 7 5 3 1

First Edition

Book design by Diane Hobbing

For Andrew,
who has shown me the beauty of second chances

Contents

Introduction

A Beautiful Connection

My older daughter, Ava, was ten when I told her I had cancer. As she struggled to understand what was happening to me, she put her feelings down on paper and wrote a poem but then hid it, too embarrassed to let me see her words. Instead, she showed it to a dear friend and colleague of mine, Sara Haines. Sara and I first met and worked together at NBC, and now we're lucky enough to work side by side at ABC. We've shared a lot of ups and downs over the years, and she's become like a sister to me and an aunt to my daughters. Sara encouraged Ava to give me the poem. She said, "Your mom needs to read this." And she was right.

Ava ran up to me one evening in the middle of my chemo treatments and handed me the neatly folded sheet of lined paper.

"Mom, please don't read this in front of me," she said as she hurried off to her bedroom and closed the door.

As I began to read Ava's words, I was overcome with pride. My little girl had so much compassion in her beautiful heart; her empathy and optimism leapt off the paper. The title of the poem was perfect, simple, and powerful: "Better." What a hopeful word. It stared back at me at a time when I felt the opposite. I was weak, but my daughter knew that I would be strong again. My tears started flowing. The voice of my ten-year-old astounded me as I marveled at her incredible wisdom. Her poem was a message of understanding and encouragement, from daughter to mother.

"Better" by Ava McIntosh

As she walks through the door with her head held up high
And a sparkle in those big blue eyes
That smile is contagious and I don't know why.
This is her battle, yet she strengthens me.
This is her struggle, and she can't be free.
This is her worry, but I have no doubt
She will survive without one pout.
She will be strong, stronger than ever.
She's a fighter just like her daughter
It has to get worse before it gets better . . .
and trust me it will get better.

My younger daughter, Annalise, was only seven when she had to hear that her mommy had cancer. She spoke to me through her art, drawing me as a princess, as if to make me all-powerful. But at the same time, I noticed how she held on to me a little tighter than before, and I could see in her big brown eyes how much she needed me.

My daughters made me rise up in my darkest moments. I felt stronger, *better,* just knowing they believed I could conquer this horrible disease. I've come to recognize that there is no clearer mirror in the world than the reflection of yourself through your children.

Despite the fact that millions of women share this awful illness, cancer can feel very isolating. I've found over this past year that every time I share my story, other women share theirs, and a beautiful connection is made. It's been a tremendous source of comfort for me, and it's the reason I decided to write this book. As a journalist, I'm much more interested in telling the story than in *being* the story. But the fact is, I didn't really have a choice about going public with my illness—I was tested on live television as a public service, and keeping quiet about the rest of my experience just felt wrong. My passion for journalism is rooted in the notion that by providing information we become stronger, more connected people. My goal is to share not only the daily challenges I faced as a newly diagnosed cancer patient but also the evolution that occurred as I transitioned from patient to survivor . . . to thriver. I am a different woman than I was before cancer. I am a better mother, wife, daughter, sister, and friend, and I've learned so much about myself. Perhaps the biggest lesson was one that I thought I knew yet too often forgot: The truth is, all I really need is exactly what I have right now.

Better

Chapter One

You Want Me to Do *What*?

I've never been a big believer in fate. Too many awful things happen to too many wonderful people for me to accept that there's a larger plan for "the greater good." But that said, I have to admit, the events that led to my diagnosis all felt very fated.

I have so many reflections that begin with *what if* and *thank God*. *What if* I had stayed at my previous job at NBC and never switched to ABC? *Thank God* I jumped networks. *What if* I hadn't become a larger part of the *Good Morning America* family, which happened only because of an unexpected twist in *GMA* host Robin Roberts's second cancer battle? I'd filled in for Robin every other week for nearly a year while she was on leave for a bone marrow transplant to fight myelodysplastic syndrome. *Thank God* I was the one who got to step in. If these things hadn't happened, I might never have received the email that ultimately saved my life.

IT WAS LATE September 2013. I was in the rural Pennsylvania home of Marie Monville, a sweet, pretty young mother of three whose husband had walked into a quiet Amish schoolhouse seven years earlier and gunned down ten little girls, killing five of them and then himself. Marie had written a memoir about her life before and after the shooting, and we were about to do her first network-television interview for ABC News. She had remarried, but she still lived in Amish Country. My producer, Kaitlyn Folmer, and I had driven out the night before and stayed at the Hotel Hershey, a few miles from Kaitlyn's childhood home. It's stunningly beautiful country, with horse-drawn carriages and pastoral farms—the last place you'd expect to find such a tragedy.

On the morning of the interview, I was still fine-tuning my questions and follow-ups as the crew finalized their camera positions and lighting. They placed Marie in front of the stone fireplace, and when I saw her there, I was struck by how incongruous it all seemed. This poised young woman in this pleasant house in bucolic Middle America had gone through a hell I couldn't begin to understand.

We were about to start rolling when I glanced at my cellphone and saw a cryptic message from *Good Morning America* producer Sandra Aiken: "Can you call me? I have a delicate assignment I need to talk to you about."

Standing in Marie Monville's kitchen, I dialed into what we call the *GMA* rim, and when I was transferred to Sandra she seemed just the slightest bit flustered. "We're going big for breast cancer awareness next month," she said. "We're going to 'Go Pink' in a major way, and we want to show women having live mammograms in our mammovan in Times Square." She paused. "We'd also like to have a member of our *GMA* team participate, and we'd like you to be that anchor."

My reaction was visceral. *No way, no how. Never gonna happen,* I thought. I knew that on-air medical screenings by members of the media, like Katie Couric's colonoscopy on the *Today* show in 2000, raised awareness and saved lives. But Katie had a personal connection to colon cancer. Her husband Jay Monahan had succumbed to the disease, and she wanted to demystify a lifesaving test that many people avoid because it's scary and uncomfortable. This was different. I've always prided myself on authenticity in my work, and this wasn't a genuine personal cause for me.

"Sandra, I don't think this is something I'm prepared to do," I said. "I've never had a mammogram before, so to have my first in front of millions of people isn't ideal."

"I understand completely," she said. "Let's talk about it when you get back to the city. Can you hold off on a decision until then?"

I agreed to that much, but nothing more.

THE INTERVIEW WAS as intense and emotional as I'd imagined it would be. Just a few years earlier, Marie had enjoyed what must have looked like a perfect life, with beautiful children and a loving husband. But then she had a miscarriage, which seemed to affect her husband even more than it did her. He blamed God, and so he decided to take it out on God's people—the Amish. She told us about the day he made a special effort to run out to the bus stop to say "goodbye" and "I love you" to their children. Only later would she realize why. This was the morning he had planned to execute his rampage. He had already purchased the ammunition and the rope to tie up his victims.

After reliving all this with Marie, I was glad to have the three-hour drive back to the city to decompress. Thinking about those schoolgirls made me want to run home to mine. I was once again reminded how lucky I was to have my family, my life, and my job. Which is when I remembered Sandra's call.

As Kaitlyn drove, I called my husband and my mom and talked it out with them. My main concern was that it might be seen as exploitative or "stunt-ish." I was afraid I would take heat from my colleagues and other media outlets for being part of a story that didn't feel like it had much to do with me. I also imagined how vulnerable I would feel with millions of people watching me do something every other woman on the planet does only in the privacy of her doctor's office. I didn't want to expose myself, literally *or* figuratively. They both agreed that having a mammogram on live TV was probably not a good idea. Then I decided to call my longtime agent and friend, Henry Reisch.

"Henry, you're never going to believe the phone call I just got," I said, and blurted it all out.

"Whoa. I was not expecting that," Henry said. "Are you going to do it?"

I quickly answered, "Well, I don't want to, but I'm calling you to figure out if that's the right answer."

Henry suggested he ask around his office to see what the reaction was and we could go from there.

I was willing to listen to a few unbiased opinions, but my mind was made up. I had every intention to politely pass on this particular assignment.

THE NEXT MORNING was Friday, September 27, and Sandra was waiting for me when I walked off the set. "Can we talk?" she asked.

I was filling in for Josh Elliott, *GMA*'s news anchor, who was in Afghanistan. Filling in was a large part of my job at the time, serving as the news division's utility infielder. If anyone from *Good Morning America* was off, I was on. If a host was missing, I hosted. If a newsreader was away, I read the news. Wherever there was a hole, I plugged it.

At the time, I had a temporary dressing room on the second floor of our Times Square offices, just above the studio where we broadcast *GMA*. Each of the anchors has a sanctuary where we prepare for the show, get our hair and makeup done, and speed-read a half dozen or so newspapers and our scripts. Sandra walked me up to mine, closed the door behind us, and explained why the producers had chosen *me* for this assignment.

"You're forty," she said. "And you've never had a mammogram. That puts you right in the middle of the demographic we're hoping to reach."

"Well, not only have I not had a mammogram," I said, "but I purposefully lost the prescription for it that my doctor wrote me a year ago." I made air quotes when I said "lost."

As soon as my ob-gyn had handed it to me the previous October, I stuck the prescription in my purse and forgot about it. Every now and then, as I was digging in my bag for my wallet or my keys, I would find that crumpled piece of paper and feel a pang of guilt for not scheduling the test. Eventually, it conveniently disappeared, probably thrown out with receipts and gum wrappers. I could say that, between my job and my kids, I was simply too busy, but the blunt truth was that I just didn't want to deal with it. Sitting there with Sandra, I still didn't feel like I *needed* a mammogram.

Sandra's eyes lit up. "That is exactly why you have to do this!"

I wasn't convinced, but I agreed to think about it a little more.

After Sandra left my dressing room, my day was far from over. It's my job to stick around and be ready to go on the air in the event of breaking news big enough for us to interrupt regular programming. I also have to update the show for the West Coast if anything changes or develops between the time we go live in the East and when we air out West.

There was no breaking news, so I was answering emails when I saw one from ABC's executive editorial producer, Santina Leuci. "If you get a mammogram in the mammovan, I will, too," it said. "Promise. Let's do it together." Santina is a force at ABC News. She is in charge of booking all the big newsmakers for the network and she essentially works 24/7, keeping us competitive. I laughed as I read the email. I could see it was not going to be easy to keep saying no.

Actually, I was starting to warm up to the idea, but first I wanted to talk to Robin Roberts, a breast cancer survivor—though she prefers the term "thriver"—to see what she thought about all of this. Robin's dressing room was just a few steps from mine. I knocked on her door, the one with the ROBIN'S NEST sign on it, and she said, "Come in."

She had already changed into her sweatpants and hoodie. Nobody is too formal coming and going from the studio—it's more like yoga pants, tank tops, and jeans. I was still in my skirt and high heels, which at least meant that I was eye-to-eye with her. (Robin is five foot ten; I'm five five.)

Her space was always dimly lit and inviting, but I wanted to make this quick. Though she'd always been cordial, we hardly knew each other. I'd been at ABC for over a year but in large part filling in for Robin, and she'd been back full-time for about a month. In September she'd passed the one-year anniversary of the stem cell transplant she underwent to treat bone marrow cancer, a disease she'd developed as a side effect of chemo.

"You're a breast cancer survivor," I started. "And I know that it's an important cause for you. . . ." I hesitated for a moment, but then I remembered how gracious she'd always been, the notes she'd sent to congratulate me on interviews I'd done. "They asked me to do a mammogram on live television on October first," I blurted out.

She laughed and said, "Oh, *you're* the one they asked!"

"That's right. Lucky me."

"I'm glad. I think you're a good choice."

"That's funny, because I don't feel that way at all. But maybe you can talk me into it. I have no connection to the disease," I explained, "so it just doesn't seem right. I mean, if my mom had had breast cancer, or if I had a sister or grandmother who'd gone through it, I'd feel like there was a reason to choose me. I'm afraid it's going to look like I'm trying to grab the limelight. I don't want to distract from the message."

Robin looked at me with a clear kindness that put me at ease. She asked, "How old are you?"

"Forty."

"And you've never had a mammogram."

"Nope."

"Amy, that's the whole point. Listen. Nobody knows better than I do how uncomfortable it can be having people watching you go through something medical. But the power of saving even one life is so remarkable, you'll never regret it." She paused, then smiled her amazing smile. "And I can pretty much guarantee it *will* save a life. Just by you walking into that mammovan and demystifying this test, someone will find out they have cancer who wouldn't have otherwise."

I was running out of objections. "But with no family history . . ."

"Amy, eighty percent of women who have breast cancer have no family history."

That's when I got the chills. I get chills a lot, and they usually serve as my internal barometer, forecasting my next move. And that statistic sent a wave from my head to my toes.

"I didn't know that," I said.

"See! You can share that, too. You can be that person. You can say, *Hey, look, I don't have a family history, I'm forty, I feel healthy, I'm going to do this anyway. I'm going to do this for me; I'm going to do this for my kids. I'm going to do this for my family.*"

Now I was nodding. Such is the power of Robin Roberts.

"I totally understand if you don't want to," she said. "And I support you either way. But I just want you to think about it in those terms."

For a moment I thought I was going to cry, but then I laughed instead. I was surprised at how emotional I was. On some level, I must have known this was a watershed moment.

"Can I give you a hug?" I said. "You just made up my mind. In fact, you made it easy."

"Sure," she said, and I gave her a big squeeze. I knew I'd made the right decision, because it felt right. A weight had been lifted off me, the pressure relieved.

I went back to my dressing room and sent an email to Sandra, saying I'd do the mammogram, but I added one request. I asked if I could tape a message to air right before the procedure, explaining why I'd agreed to do the test on live TV.

I still felt like I had to explain myself, perhaps even defend my decision, and here's why: I had spent nearly twenty years busting my butt, working eighteen-hour shifts, flying all over the world at a moment's notice, and giving up my weekends and vacations for this career, and *I was afraid to make a mistake.* I was terrified that someone would think I was insincere—because until my conversation with Robin, I didn't really believe I needed a mammogram, and to go on live television and encourage every woman my age to do a test that I had no prior intention of taking felt false. I wanted to be as up front as possible.

Once I'd made the decision, I put it all aside and spent a gorgeous fall weekend with my family at our home in the Hudson Valley, about an hour and a half north of the city. On Monday, Kaitlyn, *GMA* producer Anna Wild, and I took a crew out to do "woman on the street" interviews. "When do you think you should get your first mammogram?" we asked. It was unbelievable. No one knew. Their guesses were all over the place: fifty, thirty-five, thirty, twenty-five.

I asked, "How often should you get one? Every year? Every two years? Every five years?" Again, no one knew! Suddenly I was glad that we were going to inform women all over the country and maybe even change a few lives.

We went to the Roger Smith Hotel in Midtown to shoot my announcement. We thought the intimacy and the soft lighting of a hotel suite, rather than a sleek studio, would better capture what I wanted to say. The photographer was Russ Marhull, who's a fantastic artist and a great human being. We knew he would capture the perfect visual tone.

I jumped right in, unscripted, and hoped it would be a sincere introduction to the live segment of my procedure. "When ABC producers called me last week and asked me to have a mammogram on live national television, my first instinct was, 'No way. Never gonna do it,'" I said. Russ took a tighter shot. "I'm forty years old. I've never had a mammogram. I've avoided it, and I started thinking, *Wow, if I've put it off, how many other people have put it off, as well?* I went in to see Robin . . . and she said, 'Amy, if one life is saved because of early detection, it's all worth it.' So, Robin, this one's for you." I ended with a smile.

It's haunting to watch that clip today and to hear myself say those words before I knew that the life I saved would be my own.

TUESDAY, OCTOBER 1, the first official day of Breast Cancer Awareness Month, would be warm and sunny, but I was up long before daylight.

My usual routine was, and still is, to wake up at four, take a shower, and get dressed while my husband, two daughters, and stepson, Wyatt, are all sound asleep. We were living on Prince Street at the time, in a downtown neighborhood called NoLIta—North of Little Italy—and adjacent to SoHo—South of Houston. It's a busy area, filled with tourists, restaurants, and boutiques, and even at 4:30 A.M. when I walked out to the car, there were usually people on the street, still up from the night before. *Good Morning America* sent a car to pick me up, and because my commute took place while most people were dreaming, we could usually get to Times Square in less than ten minutes.

I had a hair and makeup team help get me camera-ready by 6:20 A.M., since every time I filled in as news anchor (like that morning) I had to do all the teases for ABC affiliates across the country, telling them what was coming up and trying to get viewers to join the *GMA* broadcast. Leading up to airtime, I spoke to local anchors in Philly and Pittsburgh and Boston and Detroit—about fifteen different cross talks in all.

I did my first news report at seven. At the top of the second hour, Robin announced, "We're hearing the word 'stronger,' and you are being so strong today, Amy Robach." She turned to me. "You're going to go live and have a mammogram. You've never had that before."

"I'm forty, I'm the age, and I have been putting it off," I said. We were only minutes away from the segment, but first I had to get through the eight o'clock news. I covered the government shutdown—the first in seventeen years—Pope Francis modernizing the Catholic Church, and falling gas prices, eventually ending on a feel-good kicker: the story of a surfer who heroically freed a loggerhead turtle from a potentially deadly fishing line.

Then we headed out to the mobile clinic in Times Square, where breast cancer survivors lined the streets. While I prepared to enter the mammovan, my PSA-like piece aired. I stepped in with my heart pounding, and there was Santina Leuci. As promised, she had gotten her mammogram. As she left the van, just out of sight of the cameras, she flashed her boobs at me. Yes, that's our beloved, crazy, brilliant Santina. She knew exactly what to do to break the tension. I'm not sure if I ever thanked her for that—so, thank you, Santina, for cracking me up when I needed it most.

I took off my pink blazer and put on a pink hospital gown. Earlier, I actually had to sign some paperwork, because this wasn't just a TV segment; this was the real deal. I had to indicate where the films were going to be sent and my ob-gyn's preference for either 3-D or 2-D imaging.

Thanks to Santina, I walked up to the mammography machine with a big smile on my face. The cameras were strategically placed, shooting me from behind and streaming live to the country. Initially, producers had asked me to wear a microphone, but I felt that no one needed a play-by-play—it was pretty obvious what was happening.

Meanwhile, Robin and Dr. Jen Ashton, an ob-gyn and ABC's senior medical correspondent, were outside the van, discussing the importance of early detection as the live images of my procedure were broadcast. Dr. Ashton is a huge contributor to our coverage of women's health and schedules mammograms for women every day.

Robin said, "When it comes to mammograms, there are a lot of myths out there and legitimate concerns, as well."

"I think one of those is about the fear of the procedure. I hear this from women all the time," said Dr. Ashton.

Meanwhile, I was inside conquering *my* fear on live television. We had very specific time restraints, so they scanned only one breast (I honestly can't remember which one), and within minutes I was back in my blazer and stepping out of the van with a huge grin on my face.

"You did it!" cheered Dr. Ashton.

"How was it?" asked Robin.

"It hurt so much less than I thought it was going to hurt," I said. "It was nothing. My Lasik eye surgery was far more painful!" I was overjoyed to report that the anticipation was far worse than the actual test. It was uncomfortable, yes, but not nearly as bad as I'd feared. On a pain scale of one to ten, it was a two.

Robin turned to the camera. "I gotta tell you, she was so nervous this morning. She is so happy right now. I can just see the relief in your eyes."

"There are tears in her eyes," said Dr. Ashton.

"That she did it," said Robin.

And that was true. I was proud and relieved all in one. I was done. *Whew!*

Or so I thought.

ONCE WE WRAPPED, a producer came running up to me. "Hey, Amy, the technicians just mentioned you didn't complete the mammogram," she said. "Before they pack it up, would you like to do the other side?"

I was *this close* to saying, *No, thanks, I'm good, I'll do it later* (as in, five to ten years later), but I felt this nagging Catholic-schoolgirl pressure to finish what I'd started, so I walked up those steps for a second time, put my other breast in several more uncomfortable positions—not in front of the camera this time—and ten minutes later I was heading home. As far as I was concerned, the story was over. I felt positive and I hoped the segment had done some good, but, honestly, I was already mentally moving on to my next assignment.

I had plenty to occupy my mind. I was a regular on *GMA*, on air three to five times a week, filling in on set, on assignment, or live-wrapping a piece from the studio. I was also a correspondent for *World News* and *Nightline,* in addition to working on several specials for ABC's news-magazine program *20/20.* I was on call seven days a week, and I never knew what my day was going to look like, because my routine was whatever the news desk told me it was going to be— sometimes that meant getting up early one day and staying late the next.

Even though I woke at 4:00 A.M. several days a week, I rarely went to bed before 10:00 P.M. When you have three active kids in the house and a husband with a busy career, getting enough sleep is pretty much impossible. My husband, Andrew Shue, is the co-founder of Cafe-Mom, an online community and information site for mothers, and he travels a lot, so we have a tough juggling act most weeks. But we've established a fairly smooth routine when we're not traveling. In the morning, Andrew gets the kids up and ready for school, and in the afternoon, I'm on pickup duty. After-school gets complicated, because on any given day the kids have gymnastics, soccer, dance, voice, writing, and guitar lessons, which requires me to shuttle them uptown, downtown, and midtown. I usually get six hours of sleep a night, which doesn't really give me the stamina my day requires. I'm not a big nap-taker, but on Thursdays I sometimes pass out before I even know what happened. And come Friday, I am definitely a party pooper, conking out on the couch at eight o'clock while we're all watching movies. Sometimes I'm out for a full twelve hours. More often, though, I wake up at four, panicked that I've missed my alarm clock, and then mumble out loud, "Oh, thank God, it's Saturday," and go back to sleep.

OVER THE NEXT several weeks, I filed news-of-the-day stories for all ABC platforms, from a Utah woman who gave birth to a healthy baby thirty-nine days after her water broke to convicted murderer Michael Skakel's new trial and release after eleven years in prison. I also covered the christening of Kate and William's royal baby, Prince George, and a *20/20* investigation into what really goes on behind the scenes in your favorite watering hole: a "bartender confidential" special.

I wasn't terribly happy bouncing around from story to story and show to show this way, so I scheduled a meeting with then–ABC News president Ben Sherwood. On October 22, we had lunch at Bar Boulud, one of my favorite restaurants near the studio, and I told Ben I was feeling very lost. "Where do I fit in?" I asked him.

He told me not to worry. "Just be patient. We have a plan."

I wasn't entirely reassured. I'm someone who makes lists, who likes to map out what lies ahead, who is always in control. This felt like the opposite.

LATER THAT DAY, I started getting emails from my assistant, Marly Faherty, saying, "Please call me ASAP." Marly is in her early twenties, is smart and hardworking, and has a bright future at ABC. When I phoned her, she told me, "The imaging center that took your mammogram has been trying to get hold of you for days. They tracked me down."

"Oh," I said. "I guess that's the strange number that's been calling me." I never answer numbers I don't know, and I rarely listen to voicemail. I'd also *completely* forgotten about the mammogram. At Marly's insistence, though, I phoned them back.

A technician told me I needed some follow-up images. "We see an area on your right breast that requires more testing," she said.

Even then—when you would think some bells might go off—I felt no fear whatsoever. I remember thinking, *This is exactly why I didn't want to get a mammogram in the first place.* It just felt like more unnecessary work—excessive testing for no good reason. I was in complete denial that anything could be wrong, but I gave the imaging center the address to send the films to my ob-gyn.

Dr. Ilene Fischer has been my doctor since I moved to New York in

2005. She's part of Kips Bay Gynecology and is affiliated with NYU Medical Center. She delivered my second daughter, Annalise, and while I was pregnant she found a benign ovarian tumor pressing against a major artery. She'd probably saved my life, so not only did she know my medical history, I trusted her completely.

"You know, Amy," she told me over the phone, "this could just be something as simple as calcium deposits. But out of an abundance of caution, we should get you over to the NYU Cancer Center. It's going to be really annoying, because they're very thorough, but let's be extra careful. It is almost assuredly nothing."

I took Dr. Fischer at her word. Then I dragged my feet about making an appointment. I remember sitting in my office, staring at my phone, knowing I should schedule it right away, but always finding something more pressing to do. I see now that it was such a childlike response: *If I ignore it, it will go away.* Perhaps it was my way of maintaining control. Perhaps distant distress signals were starting to go off, and I was angry and scared about facing the unknown. But I knew I had to tell my mom. As you might imagine, she didn't mince words.

"Amy, you need to hang up the phone with me right now and call NYU," she said. "Do not put this off, not for one day." But I still did, and she suspected as much. She barraged me with texts, meant to annoy me into action. "Have you made your appointment, Amy?" Then she got my dad to join in—a bit weird, to be honest, to have my father asking about my mammogram—and my brother, as well (that's when it got really awkward). My mom denies instigating this familial text campaign, but I know the truth. And to her credit, it worked. I only held out for two more days before making the appointment, for October 30 at 11:15 A.M.

OCTOBER HAS ALWAYS been my favorite time of year. I love the changing leaves, cozy sweaters and boots, campfires, and pumpkin pies. We have a few autumnal traditions at the Shuebach house—that's what we call our blended family, mixing Andrew's last name with mine—and one of them is apple picking. The weekend before Halloween, we grabbed the last of the apples still clinging to the orchard trees near our home upstate. The other tradition is our Oktoberfest party, which had fallen on the previous weekend. We served beer and apple cider, sausages and sauerkraut, and our friends, family, and neighbors all joined in on the festivities. It was a fun and joyful time. I was happy and grateful to be alive. I made a conscious effort to soak it all in, because I knew the next week might be emotionally difficult. Yes, my mammogram appointment was in the back of my head (and in the pit of my stomach), but my next assignment was weighing even more heavily on me.

It was the one-year anniversary of Superstorm Sandy, and *World News Tonight* had asked me to cover the communities that were devastated by the storm. On Monday, October 28, I was out in the Rockaways in Queens, where Sandy had wiped out nearly every standing structure. Everyone in the area had lost something, and many had lost everything they owned. Sadly, one year later, little progress had been made. In the neighborhood where we were shooting, only one family had actually moved back into their home—just *one*. What made the story even more poignant was that this was a community of first responders—police and firefighters—and now they were in dire need of help. We were there to shine a light on FEMA's sluggish pace in providing any assistance for rebuilding. My heart ached as they walked me through their half-redone houses: Some could show me only the foundation where their homes had once been. We went back the next day to do a live wrap, and by the end of it, our entire crew was mentally and physically exhausted.

It was eight o'clock on Tuesday before we all met up back in the city at P. J. Clarke's, just below the Empire Hotel in Midtown, to grab some dinner and drinks. There were four of us: my two producers, Dave Meyers and Kaitlyn Folmer; Michael Corn, the executive producer of *World News Tonight* at the time; and me.

When you spend time in these types of taxing situations, where you see people in such desperate need, you have to find ways to decompress. I have incredible relationships with the people I work with in the field, because we're bonded by those shared raw moments. That night, we all had a few drinks with dinner to unwind. We chatted about work gossip and what I could do for *World News Tonight* the next evening.

The mammogram never crossed my mind until Michael asked me, "What's your schedule like tomorrow?"

I checked my calendar. "I have this stupid doctor's appointment at eleven-fifteen," I said. "But I should be back in the office no later than one." I'm sure I said "stupid" to reassure myself, as I had felt a pang of anxiety when I saw the appointment pop up. I mentally shook it off, and we agreed to continue the conversation the following day. He left, and when I went up to pay our bill, the woman behind the bar said, "Your friend already picked up the tab. But he left his credit card."

"Ah," I said. "I should probably take it and give it to him. We work together." I tucked his card into my bag, and we all called it a night.

As I approached NYU's Perlmutter Cancer Center on 34th Street the next morning, I felt a slight chill, and not because of the crisp fall air. Walking into a building with the word "cancer" above the door was all it took for my procedure, which I had convinced myself was totally innocuous, to begin to feel sinister. I wanted to get in and out as quickly as possible.

It was a modern building, bright and shiny, but I noticed immediately that many of the people in the lobby were very sick, some in wheelchairs. What really got to me, though, was the presence of a string quartet playing Bach. I knew it was supposed to be soothing and uplifting, but I felt neither. All I could think was, *There must be something really serious going on when they bring in a string quartet.* It reminded me of that scene from *Titanic* in which the musicians continue to play as the ship goes down.

I checked in at the desk and then glanced at my phone to find a text from Michael, teasing me. "Hey, Robach, where's my credit card? I don't even have my wallet. I can't even buy food!"

"I'm at this appointment," I wrote back. "I promise you'll get your credit card as soon as I get to the office."

I walked into the elevator and glanced around at the people in the tiny space with me, wondering how many of them had cancer, then pushed the thought out of my head. "Out of an abundance of caution," my ob-gyn had said. *In and out,* I told myself. I was there for one more image of my right breast, and then I was heading back to my happy (if frantic) routine.

And yet I couldn't help feeling slightly vulnerable and alone. Andrew had left early that morning for Minneapolis, to talk about a big ad deal with Target for CafeMom, and just knowing he was thousands of miles away was unsettling. I had told him about the appointment but didn't mention which day it was until he texted me early that morning from the tarmac. Before Andrew or I take off on a plane, we always send each other a text: "Taking off now, love you, will call when I land." Today he'd added, "What do you have going today?" I wrote back to tell him about my follow-up exam. Right as the door was closing, he sneaked in a final text: "Let me know how it goes, call me when you get out, love you." Even if he were in town, I wouldn't have asked him to come with me—I was a big girl and I could handle it by myself. I did my best to silence the tiny voice in the back of my head that was whispering, *What if . . . ?* as I rode up.

When I got to the third floor, I only had to wait a few minutes before the staff directed me to a small room, where I changed into a bright-pink hospital gown and slippers. The gown looked more like a robe, and they provided me with a small locker for my things—the whole experience felt a little like going to the spa. If only I'd been there to get a massage.

I sat in a small, intimate waiting room with speakers playing the kind of music you might hear in a yoga studio. The hospital was taking great pains to make us feel relaxed, but as with the string quartet, there was something unnerving about all the effort.

Several women were waiting with me, but the cast of characters kept changing as new patients came in, went in, and left. Except for me. After my screening, they didn't send me on my way. They asked me to wait, then come back in for another image. I went in for four more sessions, because each time the radiologist said, "I need a better angle," or "I need a different angle," and I'd have to contort my breast into new and more uncomfortable positions, and it was becoming downright painful.

I knew the technicians were looking at a specific area, but I honestly thought they were trying to *rule out* anything suspicious. I'd been told by so many people just how unlikely it was that something could be wrong. I kept telling myself, *Okay, so I have calcium deposits. Whatever those are . . .*

Also, one of the technicians had greeted me with "I watch you every morning," so I thought they might have been overly cautious because they knew I'd had a mammogram on television and they wanted to be above reproach. I also entertained the idea that there could be a technical glitch, something wrong with the machine. Whatever it was, they just couldn't see what they needed to see, which is why mammograms are imperfect, because they don't show everything.

After the third callback, I returned to the cozy waiting room, and this time I noticed a familiar face, a woman who, like me, was being asked to go multiple rounds. She was about my age, and she looked at me and said, "Are you nervous? I hate to say it, but I'm getting scared."

I smiled, shook my head, and replied, "Not really."

Then she said, "I know who you are."

I smiled again and said, "Well, then you know I checked the statistics on this."

She responded, "I know. I know you did a story."

"I did," I said. "Less than one percent. There's at most a one percent chance of having breast cancer at our age. How old are you?"

"I'm forty," she said. "But I don't know my family history, because I was adopted, so I'm kind of freaking out."

"Family history doesn't matter that much. The fact is, you're young, you're healthy." Then I added, "Chances are, you and I are fine. We'll laugh about this tomorrow."

She paused and then said, "I'm not sure I will. I felt a lump, and I really think I have breast cancer." I tried to think of something more to say, because her expression was so anguished.

"There are also so many false positives," I began. "You can't think like that. Focus on the statistics. Statistically speaking, you're going to be perfectly healthy."

"Thank you for saying that," she said, smiling. "I feel a little better now."

A moment later I got another text from Michael. "Hey, Robach? Are you in the building yet?"

I texted back, "I'm stuck here. I don't know what's taking so long. I'm sorry. Do you want to send your assistant down here?"

But the next time I got called in, I didn't go back to the waiting room. The technician told me that they weren't getting a clear-enough image, so she had to do a sonogram—which is the point at which my mind shifted away from my iPhone and toward what was happening to me right here, right now. This sounded serious.

Moments later, I found myself lying in a dark room with a cold steel instrument circling my breast. The radiologist kept going over and over and over one specific area. My skin became sensitive, and I closed my eyes to try to control the urge to jump off the table and scream, *Stop it!* But then I tilted my head to see what was on the screen, and the image was undeniable. The radiologist didn't need to point out what she then referred to as a "small mass." It was right there, a dark spot on the screen: a tumor about the size of a marble, growing inside me.

My mind went back to previous sonograms I'd had. They'd produced the first images of the tiny beautiful miracles growing inside me, my daughters. But this was no miracle. This was a nightmare.

The radiologist caught my eye, and then we both went back to looking at the screen. "You couldn't feel that?" she said. She took my hand and put it on my breast. "You couldn't feel that?" she repeated.

Sure enough, my two fingers were going back and forth over a lump just beneath my armpit. I had never done a self-exam, but at that moment I wished so much that I had.

I said, "Well, I feel it now." I wondered if she was actually trying to make me feel worse than I already did. And, a few seconds later, she succeeded.

"We have to do a biopsy," she said. "I'd like you to stay and do that now. Do you have time?"

"Of course," I said.

My throat tightened as I continued to stare at the tumor. I couldn't shake the stark contrast between witnessing new life versus staring down death. Tears welled up in my eyes.

I texted Andrew. "I need to talk to you, I'm getting really concerned," I wrote. "They're telling me I need a biopsy, call me ASAP." So much for the breezy text that I had anticipated sending, letting him know I was on my way back to work.

I wanted to stay positive, so I kept telling myself that this was why some people argued against forty-year-olds getting mammograms: excessive testing, false readings, unnecessary anxiety. I was sure I was living it. *It has to be benign,* I repeated over and over, as if I were saying the rosary. The statistics were heavily in my favor—99 to 1.

But there I was, alone and scared in my pink hospital gown.

In came another doctor and another nurse. They talked in hushed tones in the corner. It was like a scene from a medical drama on TV right before bad news is delivered, and it really hit me: This was definitely not good.

I had kept my phone nearby in case Andrew got in touch. I was desperate to hear his voice. It buzzed, but it was just a text from Michael's assistant. "Hey, Amy, I'm in the waiting room. I need to get that credit card." *Are you kidding me?* I thought.

Then my phone rang, but this time it was Josh Elliott. We'd become great pals during my time at ABC, and he wanted to vent about something that had happened that morning on *GMA*. I didn't want to tell him where I was, so I did my best to have a normal conversation in the middle of this very abnormal situation. The nurse started trying to get my attention.

"Ms. Robach."

"Hey, Josh, can I let you go? I've got a . . ."

"Yeah, sure. But just one more thing—"

"Ms. Robach," the nurse repeated. *This is something more than calcium deposits.*

"No, seriously, I'm at the doctor's office, and I'm getting these tests, and I've been called back about three times now, and I actually have to go. I'm sorry."

He said, "What?"

I had to hang up, and he immediately started texting me: "Are you okay? Please tell me you're okay."

But from that moment on, any reality outside that exam room was a world away. My friends, my job, and my everyday life all felt like they were someone else's as I sat on that exam table, holding my breath.

My heart was pounding, and I was thinking, *This really can't be happening.* I was still holding on to hope that they'd tell me it was just something we needed to watch, a mild cause for concern but certainly nothing life-altering. I kept telling myself, *It's not cancer.*

Yet another doctor came into the room. She was older and looked like she was in charge, and she consulted with the younger radiologist, who had performed my sonogram. The nurse in the room glanced at me now and then as they talked.

After a few minutes, the supervising doctor gave me a brief smile and nod, then left the room; the radiologist walked over to my examining table.

"We're going to do a biopsy called a fine-needle aspiration," she said. "We'll have the results in about five to ten minutes. Would you like them now, or would you like to wait until you can have someone with you?"

Who could wait when it was phrased like that? "I'm going to want them now," I said.

She brought in her instruments and explained the procedure while the nurse gently stroked my hand. Tears pooled in my eyes as I tried to process what was happening. The needle went in with some serious pressure, accompanied by the sound of a staple gun. The doctor repeated this three more times, and it was over.

She left with the sample, and almost immediately my phone rang again. It was finally Andrew. He'd been in the middle of a lunch in Minneapolis with about a dozen women, and as soon as he saw my text, he'd stepped outside to call me. I told him, "There is a mass in my right breast. I saw it in the sonogram. I'm really, really scared, Andrew." I began to cry full on.

He did his best to say the right things. "I love you, and I know it's going to be okay. Whatever happens, we will figure it out together."

"Thank you, baby. I've been trying to tell myself that it has to be benign, but now I have this awful feeling, and I'm freaking out."

Then the radiologist was back. She leaned into the room, peeking her head around the door. "Again, I just wanted to check to make sure you wouldn't rather have someone with you."

"My husband's on the line with me right now. I can put him on speaker," I said.

She nodded and disappeared again.

"I need you to wait on the phone with me," I told Andrew. "They're going to give me the results." Even though he was twelve hundred miles away, I felt safer just hearing his voice and feeling his love on the other end of the line. I needed him more than anything at that moment, especially with all the activity in the exam room. It seems as if the most dramatic events in our lives happen in slow motion, and that's exactly how I remember this unfolding—at a slow, warped, nauseating pace.

The radiologist came back with the lab report. Maybe she could see the caller ID on my phone screen, or maybe she remembered from my records, but she immediately addressed Andrew by name.

"Mr. Shue," she said. "I have your wife's biopsy results, but first I have to ask you something. *Are you driving?*"

And that's when I knew.

It was like a line out of a movie. Did doctors say things like that in real life? Well, this one did, and my throat tightened even more, and the tears streamed down my face, and I knew what was coming next.

"The tumor we found in your wife's right breast is malignant."

On Andrew's end of the line, there was nothing but silence. On my end, there was sobbing, loud sobbing.

The nurse standing next to me began to rub my back. "I hate this part of my job," she said. "I am so, so sorry." My shoulders heaved as pain coursed through my entire body.

Then, in an almost comically awkward attempt to get a response from my husband, the radiologist said, "Mr. Shue, your wife is not taking the news very well." That was an understatement. But who takes this kind of news *well*?

I took the phone off speaker and asked, "Did you hear that? Are you there?" I repeated what the doctor had just said.

Andrew said the conversation was too hard to follow on speakerphone, that "malignant" was not a word he was expecting. I could tell he was stunned.

"When are you coming home?" I asked through my tears. "I need you now. I don't know what to do next."

"I'm on my way to the airport," he said.

THERE ARE ONLY two people in our family—and it's a big Catholic family on both sides—who have had cancer at an early age. When my uncle Kevin was thirty-six, doctors discovered an astrocytoma, a malignant tumor, in his brain. He had surgery, but the tumor came back as a grade 4 glioblastoma, the most aggressive form possible. After more surgery, chemotherapy, and radiation, Uncle Kev defied all medical odds and is still alive and well today, eleven years later. But my uncle Frank's wife, my aunt Janet, was not as lucky. She died at forty-eight of non-Hodgkin's lymphoma and left three children behind in Harlan, Kentucky. I watched her fight bravely for two years and saw her deteriorate beyond recognition at the end. I was pregnant with Ava when she died. At her funeral, I was immensely moved as I watched her oldest son, Jeffrey—who was struggling, naturally—muster up enough strength to play a beautiful ballad on his guitar in her honor. The impact of her death was catastrophic, and still is today, twelve years later.

Is that what's going to happen to us? I thought. I felt sure that I was dying—that I was going to die—and I was reeling. I thought I might throw up or pass out.

After hanging up with Andrew, I felt even more alone. I needed to talk to someone else. But who is the next person you tell? Whose life do you ruin next?

I tried to compose myself, because people were looking at me as if they were surprised that I was so upset. As if I shouldn't be so upset or at least shouldn't *show* it. As if my reaction was upsetting *them.* I talked about my kids. I kept saying, "What am I going to tell my little girls?"

A nurse came over and asked, "Would you like to talk to a therapist, to help you process what's just happened? We have someone who could help you figure out how to talk to your children."

I said, "Yes, actually, I would really appreciate that." I needed someone by my side, even if it was a complete stranger.

In the meantime, I tried to call my brother, Eric, who's a doctor. I knew he'd be able to process the news as a physician (rationally and without a lot of emotion), and I desperately wanted his strength and his guidance. He could also help me with the next call I knew I had to make: my mom.

Mom and I are very close. She used to joke that if anything ever happened to my brother or me, she would have to be institutionalized. She gave up most of her personal life by having me at nineteen and my brother at twenty-one. She dropped out of college to raise us, while my dad stayed in school and built his career.

But Eric didn't answer, so I decided to bite the bullet and call Mom before I lost my nerve.

When she answered, all I could manage at first was a high-pitched cry of "Mom . . . ?" Then, after a long pause: "They found a tumor. It's malignant."

For a moment, she didn't say anything. I know she must have been shocked and panicked just like me, but she didn't let me hear it. She simply said, "Don't worry, sweetie, you're going to be okay. Dad and I are going to get on the first plane to New York. We'll be there tonight."

It was the shortest call my mom and I have ever had. We usually talk for at least forty-five minutes to an hour, easily. She told me later that she *knew* as soon as the phone rang that I had bad news. It was one of those sixth-sense moments that I believe all mothers experience.

The nurse reappeared in the room and handed me a piece of paper. "We're going to need you to meet with a surgeon," she said. I looked down at a list of names. "Do you have any idea who you'd like to see?" she asked me.

I found this utterly strange, that here in the middle of a cancer diagnosis I was supposed to go doctor-shopping. As I scanned the names through my bleary, tear-filled eyes, I tried to face the fact that one of these doctors would very likely be operating on me, and I knew nothing about any of them. How was I supposed to pick?

"Which one would you choose, if it were you?" I asked.

"I'd go with the one who could see me right now," she said.

"Okay, I'll go with that. Who's here?"

A few moments later, she walked me down to a small office with a love seat and a coffee table. While I waited to meet Dr. Deborah Axelrod, I started crying again. It all seemed so surreal. I called Kaitlyn Folmer, who in a very short period of time had become one of my dearest friends. I had been keeping her up to date via text. She was helping me deal with Michael Corn's assistant, who was still in the waiting room. But I hadn't given her the results of the biopsy yet.

"Do you want me to come?" she asked. "I can be there in fifteen minutes."

"I would actually love that. Thank you," I said. I wasn't retaining what the doctors and nurses were telling me. There were so many details, so many decisions to make. I needed someone by my side. Kaitlyn was on her way.

As soon as we hung up, the phone rang again, and it was my brother, Eric. At the sound of his voice, I blurted out the news, and he went straight into clinical mode, just as I'd hoped he would. Eric is an internist in Athens, Georgia; he's twenty months younger than I am and about the smartest person I know.

"You should consider double mastectomy," he told me. "You're only forty, Amy. You're young, and you're going to want to be as aggressive as you can be to make sure the doctors get everything and that you save yourself the hassle of constant monitoring. You do not want to be going back for mammograms every couple of months and facing more biopsies and more fear. Get rid of them and save yourself a lot of heartache." That was my brother, direct and opinionated, and I was glad for it. In that moment, his resoluteness gave me much-needed strength.

Then he brought up something that, in my addled state, I hadn't even considered. "You also have to prepare yourself mentally for chemo. I know we still have a lot to find out about your cancer, whether or not it's spread. But because of your age alone, I can almost guarantee your oncologist will be in favor of it."

I took a minute to let it all sink in, but it didn't go down in a slow, deep-inhale kind of way. It was more like gulping Drano—a raging flow of caustic information that overwhelmed my brain, then settled into my gut, thick and rancid.

I thought back to just a few hours earlier at breakfast, when I'd been trying to eat my way through the pain of cutting loose with my colleagues the night before. That was the life I wanted back, where the worst thing I had to deal with was a hangover and a growling stomach. I had planned to head straight into work after this appointment. Instead, here I was talking to my brother about surgically removing my breasts and undergoing months of debilitating treatment.

There was a knock on the door, but the doctor who entered wasn't Dr. Axelrod. It was the therapist. She was cerebral-looking, in her fifties, very sweet and calm.

I immediately asked her how to tell my young daughters the news. She said there was no need to wait or to shy away, that they might actually be more worried if I shrugged off my obvious distress and told them nothing was wrong.

"But what do I say?" I needed a line-by-line script.

"They're old enough to know that something's wrong. And if you don't tell them, they'll fill in the blanks with something worse. So be honest. Just make them feel safe. Tell them you are not going to die."

We talked it over a bit more, and I went through about half a box of Kleenex. After I'd calmed down a bit, she said, "You know, it's okay to cry. It would be strange if you didn't. But keep it simple. Tell them you have the best doctors. Tell them you're getting the best care possible. Make them feel like you're on top of it."

In a sense, she was giving me permission to do what I already knew I had to do: tell them, straight up. I knew I couldn't just walk in and say, *Hey, guys. Let's make dinner!* and pretend nothing was wrong. Kids are intuitive. But I wanted to make sure I wasn't going to do anything to scar them for life, either.

Then Dr. Axelrod came in, and I liked her immediately. She was in her fifties, trim and athletic-looking. And there was a confidence about her, maybe even a cockiness, that made me feel safe. Self-doubt is not something you want in a surgeon.

We shook hands, and then she leaned against her desk.

"I don't know what's going on today," she said. "You're the third woman in her forties who's just been diagnosed with breast cancer."

That's when I felt the chills again, because I knew the poor woman I tried to comfort in the waiting room *had* to be one of the patients she was talking about. I had told her we were going to be fine, and neither of us was.

I thought the therapist might leave, but she stayed with me as the doctor got down to business, talking about my diagnosis and plan for treatment.

"You have a tumor in your right breast, just under two centimeters. But from what we can see in the sonogram, there's no evidence your lymph nodes have been affected. The most conservative surgical approach would be a lumpectomy—"

I stopped her short. "I'm ninety-nine percent sure I want a double mastectomy," I said.

I saw her eyebrow rise ever so slightly, but what Eric had told me made sense, and I felt in my gut that this was the right thing to do. I wanted to be aggressive, and I was willing to endure the physical repercussions.

"Okay," she said, "but let's not jump to that. Your tumor isn't large, and we may have caught it early."

She glanced at the therapist. Then she said, "Let's take the decision in stages. The first thing we need is an MRI. We should be able to get you in within the hour."

A nurse came to escort me back to the waiting room once more, and when we stepped into the corridor, Kaitlyn was coming out of the elevator. She was carrying a big plastic bag from the deli downstairs.

"I figured you haven't eaten," she said, pulling out items one by one. "I got you this cup of fresh fruit, and here are some crackers in case you're feeling nauseated and Smartwater to replenish your electro-lytes." She even thought to buy a box of tissues. She opened them and handed me one. It was so sweet that I started laughing through my tears.

"We will figure this out; it's going to be okay," she said, and gave me a big hug.

At that moment, my producer became more than just a dear friend. She became the sister I never had. Now that I had someone to look after me (and make sure I was properly hydrated), the therapist wished me well and excused herself.

Kaitlyn, in her best TV-producer fashion, whipped out her note-book and pen and became my memory bank, writing down my up-coming appointments and all the decisions ahead of me. What kind of surgery should I have? Who should I choose as my oncologist?

Minutes later, a technician led us to a room dominated by a magnetic-resonance-imaging machine. I'd had an MRI before, so I knew how awful it was to be inserted into a narrow tube with only a few inches to spare and then lie perfectly still for an hour in a machine that makes insanely loud knocking sounds the entire time. But this time, the nurse explained, I would have to go through all of this lying facedown, with my breasts fitted into indentations in a tray. I couldn't believe it. I'd been crying for three hours straight, and my sinus cavity was full. There weren't enough tissues in the hospital, and now I was going to have to lie on my stomach, with the pressure of all that crying making my face throb. My hands had to stay by my sides, unable to wipe tears or other fluids falling from my face. I felt like I was in an upside-down coffin.

"I don't know if I can do this," I said. My face was puffy and red, and every five seconds another wave of tears came pouring out. But I did it, with the machine going *thunk, thunk, thunk* all the while and the thoughts in my head torturing me. *How did I get here? Is this really happening?*

After a full hour they pulled me out, and I agreed to come back in the morning to discuss the results with Dr. Axelrod. But my day wasn't over yet.

Next I had to see Dr. Julia Smith, a geneticist, whose office was a couple of blocks away. Kaitlyn had to literally take me by the hand and lead me down the street. At this point I'd seen five doctors, maybe six, and I was a total wreck. Aside from the few pieces of fruit that Kaitlyn brought me, I hadn't eaten anything since breakfast. I had walked into NYU at 11:15 A.M., and now it was almost five o'clock. My eyes were practically sealed shut from all the crying. I felt light-headed and dizzy, and I'm pretty sure I looked like a zombie from my personal TV obsession, *The Walking Dead,* as we made our way down Lexington Avenue.

Fortunately, Dr. Smith was exactly the person I needed to meet at that moment. She had a warm smile and was incredibly positive and maternal. She was tiny, with gray hair and lots of energy—like a cool grandma—and I felt an instant connection.

She took my hand and said, "You're going to be okay. We're going to make sure that you and I know each other for a very long time." Which is when I started to cry all over again, but this time it was because she was saying what I needed to hear—reassuring me that my life wasn't over, that whatever I might have to go through, I was still going to be around. "Forty-year-olds are not supposed to get breast cancer," she went on. "So we have to figure out why this happened to you. Clearly something went wrong, whether it was environmental or genetic. You're the exact kind of person I want to study."

Then she asked me a lot of questions. How often did I exercise? How much did I drink? Did I have any Jewish blood in my family?

"Not that I know of," I said.

"I still want to have you tested. It might be a bit of a fight with the insurance company, but this is important information for you to have, especially as the mother of two daughters. BRCA1 and BRCA2 are the genes we're worried about. They produce proteins that suppress tumors. If you have mutations in those genes, your cell replication isn't as stable, and DNA damage may not be repaired properly. As a result, cells are more likely to develop additional genetic alterations that can lead to cancer. Certain populations have higher rates of mutation in these genes: Ashkenazi Jews, Norwegians, Dutch, Icelanders. . . ."

She typed some information into her computer and said, "There are a lot of things you can do, depending on your course of action. You'll need to cut back on alcohol. And I'd like you to limit your red-meat intake to about once or twice a month at most." Although I'd been through much worse that day, that stung. I'm a Midwestern girl. I'll admit I love red meat. "But don't worry," she said. "That mammogram just saved your life. If you'd been diagnosed with this ten years ago, you would have had a completely different course of treatment. So imagine where we're going to be ten years from now."

Kaitlyn, who'd been writing all this down, gave me a smile. It was the first glimmer of hope I'd felt all day.

Then Dr. Smith said, "Go home and have a glass of wine. We can talk more about alcohol intake later."

And with that, my long and emotionally exhausting day at the hospital was over. Kaitlyn and I went outside, hailed a cab, and headed downtown.

Chapter Two

"I Promise, I'm Not Going to Die"

As Kaitlyn and I rode down Second Avenue, my new reality continued to wash over me in waves of nausea and anxiety. It all seemed so surreal, so impossible. One thing I knew for certain was that I wouldn't talk to my children without Andrew by my side. But it would still be another hour or so before he even landed at LaGuardia.

We had the driver stop on Prince Street, outside my neighborhood French café. It was a block away from my apartment, and Kaitlyn agreed to wait with me until Andrew could meet us. My daughters would be spared the news for a little while longer.

It was now 6:00 P.M. and getting dark, but New Yorkers don't eat until 8:00, so we were the only people in the restaurant. We ordered the special, split pea soup, and two glasses of rosé.

At that moment, I was filled with gratitude for Kaitlyn. In fact, I'm always thankful for Kaitlyn. She was assigned to anchor-produce for me when I subbed for Robin, and we hit it off immediately. She is a major force in the unlikeliest of bodies: less than one hundred pounds and just over five feet tall. She was adopted as an infant from South Korea and raised in Amish Country. Kaitlyn is the kind of person who will drop everything at a moment's notice to chase a story and won't stop until she brings home the prize—all while wearing five-inch designer heels. She's insanely organized and makes these incredible binders (I've tweeted pictures of them, they're so epic) filled with more information about a given story than you could ever absorb. Packing those binders, which weigh fifteen to twenty pounds, is never easy, but it's always worth it when I'm cramming for an interview on a flight. Whether I'm covering Boko Haram kidnappings in the middle of Nigeria or waiting for a royal birth outside St. Mary's Hospital in London, Kaitlyn is there, making sure I have all the information I need. And right then, what I needed most was a friend.

How was I going to tell my kids? The therapist had stressed how important it was to make them feel safe, but safe was the last thing *I* felt. I couldn't stop thinking about how young my daughters were and how much time I needed on this earth to guide them and love them. Graduations, weddings, and grandchildren all flashed in front of me. My heart ached at the thought of missing those big moments and all the little ones in between.

I thought about my first experience with serious illness. When I was growing up in St. Charles, Missouri, my best friend since first grade, Stacey Schneider, battled leukemia. She was diagnosed in second grade and had to go through intense chemotherapy. Eventually she lost all of her brown wavy hair and wore a navy-blue-and-white bandanna around her head. While the other kids ran around the big parking lot the school used as our playground, we'd just sit together on the curb and talk, because she was usually too tired to jump rope or play hopscotch.

By third grade, she was permanently hospitalized, and that fall our teacher had each of the kids in our class tape-record a message for her. When it was my turn, I sat in the supply closet (our "sound booth"), pressed RECORD, and told her what our class was doing, how much I missed her, and how I hoped she would feel better soon. When she died the following spring, I was asked to give one of the Bible readings at her funeral. I was only nine, but I wanted to be brave for Stacey, so I stood in front of the congregation and read a short passage from the Old Testament. After the funeral mass at our church was over, the adults—including my parents—continued on to the burial, but I went back to school. Mom and Dad thought the cemetery would be too much for me to witness. Back in the classroom, I looked out the window and saw a gigantic bright rainbow filling up the entire sky. One of the nuns ran in and said, "Look, children, a gift from Stacey. She's sending us a big smile in the sky." At the time I was filled with joy, but later that night, after my mom had tucked me into bed and turned out the lights, the thought that Stacey could communicate from the dead haunted me. I couldn't sleep. My heart pounded. After breaking out in a sweat, I got out of bed and sat at my little desk to write Stacey a letter. It said, "I miss you and love you. I saw your beautiful rainbow today, and I hope heaven is great, but please don't come see me." I went back to bed, feeling relieved. *She's going to read that,* I thought, *and she's not going to wake me up. It's all going to be okay.*

Death is a difficult concept for any child, and so is a serious illness that can lead to death. My daughters were roughly the same age as I had been when Stacey was sick, and I knew that to watch somebody who's strong suddenly become weak and vulnerable can be very frightening. A best friend was bad enough. But your mom?

I looked out the window at all the people going about their normal business: walking their dogs, laughing with friends, heading out for the night. This was when I'd normally be winding down, and I remembered that I was supposed to be at work at five the next morning—in costume as Princess Kate, for our Halloween show. There was no way I could act like a proud new royal mommy twelve hours from now, in front of six million people.

I called Barbara Fedida, ABC's senior vice president for talent and business. Barbara was the one who'd first reached out to bring me over to ABC from NBC. She called me even before she was officially announced at ABC, to see if I was willing to consider making the network switch. We had met seven years earlier, when she was at CBS, and had always plotted to work together one day. She's the person you go to when you have an issue. Sadly, the network had gained far too much experience dealing with issues like mine. In 2005, *World News Tonight* anchor Peter Jennings died of lung cancer. Then, in 2007, Joel Siegel, *GMA*'s beloved film critic, succumbed to colon cancer. And, of course, Robin Roberts had battled breast cancer and then bone marrow cancer.

Barbara was on a plane, about to leave Miami. "The doors are closing," she said. "Can I call you back when I land?"

"This can't wait," I said. But even then I found myself hesitating, unable to get the words out. *Rip off the Band-Aid,* I thought. *Do it quickly.* "I had a follow-up mammogram today and found out I have breast cancer."

Barbara was silent for a moment, then said, "Amy, I am so sorry." She stayed with me on the line, incredibly supportive, asking for details, asking how I felt. Later, she told me she almost got kicked off the plane for not shutting down her cellphone.

Barbara had a three-hour flight to process our phone conversation, and as soon as she landed in New York she sent an email to *GMA*'s executive producer, Tom Cibrowski, explaining why I wouldn't be on the show the next day.

And then there were other calls I had to make. One of the hardest was to my former husband, Tim McIntosh, who lives just north of the city in Bronxville and is the father of my two daughters. As soon as he heard my voice, he immediately said, "It's your grandmother, isn't it?" Tim and I met when we were nineteen. We were engaged at twenty-two and married at twenty-three. He knew my family about as well as his own.

"No," I said. "It's me."

"What do you mean?"

"I found out today I have breast cancer."

"Oh, God, Amy. I'm so sorry."

"I'm going to tell the girls tonight. I can't hide it, and they're old enough to know. So please be there for them. I know how much you love them and want to be strong for them. I need you to be their rock and to help them feel safe. You've got to reassure them and let them know they can talk to you about anything, at any time. If there's anything they can't say to me, I want them to say it to you."

"Absolutely," he said. There was a long silence, and then he added, "Let me know if there's anything I can do, Amy."

My next call from the little French café was to Henry, my agent. He listened to my news, took a deep breath, and said, "Thank God you got that mammogram."

We both paused, and I thought about just how close I'd come to not having it. Then Henry switched modes from agent to friend. "What can I do? What do you need from me? Who's your physician? I know people, so let me know if you don't like your doctor. Have you made any decisions about surgery?"

Henry is about ten years older than me, and he's always played a big-brother role in my life. As we said goodbye, he said, "Wait a minute, I have to tell you something. I love you, Amy."

I started crying again, but I pulled myself together, because I had yet another call to make. Kaley, my babysitter, had only been with us since the beginning of the school year—just two months—but the kids loved her. She was twenty-two and she had her own apartment in Brooklyn, but she was always there for us, running around the city when I couldn't be in three different places at one time, picking up Wyatt from track, Ava from voice, and Anna from gymnastics. Kaley was my logistics girl, helping get the kids to school when Andrew and I were traveling and then with the afternoon runaround. Sometimes she'd spend the night with us or show up at four in the morning. Andrew and I always try to be at drop-offs and pickups and as many activities as possible, but Kaley's most important job was simply to be there when we couldn't, and this was one of those times.

She was helping the girls with their homework when I called. "Kaley, can you step away from the kids right now?"

"Sure," she said. "What is it?"

I felt bad, because I'd told her I was going to be home by four or five at the latest. I'd been texting her since three: "Hey, I'm stuck getting tests at the doctor's. I haven't been able to leave yet." And now it was after six o'clock.

Even though I had already said it out loud several times, telling my babysitter I had cancer still felt unreal, like some kind of out-of-body experience. She was speechless. I felt awful for making her so uncomfortable.

"I'm going to be home soon," I said. "I'm actually only a block away, waiting for Andrew, and then we're going to come home and tell the kids. Can you help them have a little bit of fun before I have to break the news? Why don't you order some pizza and rent a movie, maybe pop some popcorn."

"Of course," she said.

It was just after 7:00 p.m. when Andrew walked into that café on Prince Street, still carrying his bags. My face was so puffy and tear-stained that I was thankful the candlelight was dim and he could barely see me.

"That was the longest three-hour flight I've ever had," he said, and wrapped his arms around me and whispered, "Oh, baby, it's going to be okay." I buried my face in his neck. I pride myself on being tough and independent, but I needed to be held. I love the way my husband smells, and for that moment it seemed possible that everything *would* be okay. But I knew Andrew was panicked. I could see the strain on his face. He'd lost his father to cancer only five months before and was still having a hard time coping. We sat there for a few minutes as I filled him in on the doctors I'd met, what they'd said, and what our day looked like tomorrow. Andrew and I held hands under the table, buying a little more time before heading home.

When we got up to leave, I gave Kaitlyn a big, long hug.

"I couldn't have made it without you today," I said.

"I was just glad I could be there," she replied.

Now it was time to face my children. I'll never forget that walk down Prince Street: the tourist-filled sidewalks, the cupcake bakeries, the boutiques filled with the latest fashions. It didn't seem possible that there was a tumor inside me, threatening my life. I didn't feel any different. I didn't feel sick—I wasn't even tired. I had no symptoms whatsoever, and here I was on this beautiful October night with my husband, on this familiar street where everyone was bustling and laughing and drinking wine in the outdoor cafés. Andrew and I held hands as we slowly made our way, both in a gauzy stupor, toward number 40, our second-floor loft, and our waiting children.

When we got to the door, Ava and Annalise rushed me, almost knocking me over with hugs.

"Mommy, Mommy . . . where have you been?" they squealed, and with that, my tears started flowing again.

I relished having those little arms around me, all the more so because of what I had to tell them and because I knew the effect it was going to have on them. Their world was never going to be the same.

I wish I could have been more stoic, more guarded, but that's just not who I am. My friends always tease me that everyone in the room can tell exactly what I'm thinking, so I'd never make much of a poker player. Ava was ten at the time, Annalise was seven, and my stepson Wyatt was ten, and they'd never seen me quite like this before. Even though I was able to take a few breaths and control my tears, I could feel my lips shaking.

I said, "Mommy has had a really tough day, and I need to talk to you guys." I put my arms around them and we walked toward the couch. Our open space had seen a lot of joy over the past year. When we decided to rent the loft, we joked that it was the perfect apartment to throw a party in, and we did, many, many times. We'd had dancing, DJs, and a karaoke machine in that loft. We had already hosted two baby showers, parties for the Super Bowl and for Halloween. Was this the end of the good times?

The girls fell around me like kittens, crowding out Wyatt, who sat down in a chair next to me. Andrew was on the couch next to us.

"What I'm about to tell you is going to be really hard to hear, but I need you to know this first—I am going to be okay." I took a deep breath and said, "I've been at the hospital all day because the doctors found a tumor in my breast—and it is cancer."

Ava burst into tears. She's like me in that she carries her emotions in plain sight, and the word "cancer" was enough to set off a crying binge. Annalise, my little one, seemed to go inward instead. I don't think she knew how to react, so she simply squeezed my arm and buried her head in my chest. Seeing her big sister so upset, she also began to cry but more quietly. My stepson Wyatt, usually so cuddly, squirmed in the chair next to me and covered his face with his hands.

I tried to fill the void with explanations. "The doctors are going to take the tumor out very soon. It's not going to be fun, but I'm going to live. I promise, I'm not going to die."

I tried to be reassuring, repeating the things the doctors had told me: *The tumor's not that big. I'm going to have surgery very soon.* As I rubbed their backs, their sobbing slowly grew softer. We held one another for what seemed like an hour. I could tell they were afraid to let me go, squeezing me so hard that, although it felt good, it also felt scary. I tried to inject a little humor. I told them about the possibility of chemotherapy, and I explained that I might lose all my hair.

"So who's going to shave their head with me?" I said.

The girls both looked at me. "Not us," they said, and then we all started laughing, though for Ava it was still through tears.

"Oh, really?" I said, feeling myself smile for the first time in hours. "You love me, but you're not going to shave your head for me. Okay. If that's the way it's going to be."

Andrew stepped away to call his two older sons, Aidan and Nate, then seventeen and fifteen, who were at boarding school in New Jersey about an hour outside the city. They'd just lost their grandfather, and Nate asked the question of the day: "Why does this keep happening?"

It was a sobering comment, but luckily it was followed almost immediately by my parents' arrival. I breathed a deep sigh of relief as they came through that door and wrapped me in their arms. My dad had come straight from work. He was wearing a suit and carrying his briefcase.

My mom had walked in with a look of love and fear on her face, but she was strong for my children as they ran to their grandparents for big hugs and kisses. They love their Noanie and Pop, and watching my girls with my parents, I felt calm for the first time since I'd walked into that doctor's office. The truth is, they had me when they were so young—only nineteen—they could pass for Ava and Anna's parents.

"Isn't this exciting?" I said, as brightly as I could. "Noanie and Pop made it just in time to go trick-or-treating with us! They get to be here for our favorite holiday."

We had plans to go up to Tim's neighborhood in Bronxville the next evening, because trick-or-treating in New York City doesn't feel quite right. Going door-to-door in an apartment building isn't nearly as fun as running from house to house on a decorated block with the crisp October air all around you.

"Sounds good," my mom said. "But tomorrow we have to go shopping! I have no idea what I packed, and I'm pretty sure I forgot most of my toiletries. I don't even know what clothes I have." She'd thrown whatever was closest into a suitcase and run out the door to meet my father at the airport.

We were all trying not to show any fear, and the look on my parents' faces was so loving it broke my heart. I realized how much more scared I would be if one of my children had cancer instead of me. That's what my parents were living through right now—the worst-case scenario. But they were being so brave. I was desperate to feel grounded and contained, and with them there, and all of us together, I finally felt some security.

It was past the time to get Ava, Anna, and Wyatt to bed. Everyone was mentally exhausted, so there was little complaining: The kids all slept in the boys' room, where we had bunk beds and a trundle. My parents would stay in my daughters' room.

Our apartment had a small sitting area just outside the bedrooms. My parents and Andrew huddled around me, and we dimmed the lights and had a glass of wine as we went over the next steps. We had to whisper so we wouldn't wake the kids, which fit the mood: surreal, even a little spooky. I was scared as hell.

My follow-up appointment with Dr. Axelrod was at ten the next morning, and my mom and dad planned to come with Andrew and me after we dropped off the kids at school. We talked about how we could distract the kids over the next couple of days. My parents swore they wouldn't leave my side until we had a long-term plan. I can't remember how I got to sleep that night. Maybe I took an Ambien, or maybe I simply collapsed, but somehow I managed to sleep until six-thirty.

When you first wake up after something devastating happens, there's a moment when you can trick yourself into believing it was all a dream. But in the bright morning light, there was no escaping my new unreality: I had cancer. I was a cancer patient.

Despite looking like the picture of health, I was all those things that previously applied only to *other* people—people with no hair, people who were thin and weak and sickly. It just didn't seem possible.

Fortunately, I didn't have much time to dwell on it. I had to help the kids get ready for their Halloween festivities at school. The one tiny silver lining to this horrible cloud was that after all my years of travel and early wake-up calls, I was home to help them on one of the most fun days of the year.

Annalise was the only one who really had to be made up, because she was going to school in full costume as a princess, and she was super-excited. Ava and Wyatt were in the upper school and considered too big for the full regalia, so for them today was simply Crazy Hat Day—much easier. Before we left the apartment, I wrote an email to each of their teachers explaining that my children had just found out that their mom had cancer. I asked them to please let me know if they saw any evidence of the kids being upset or withdrawn.

Then we all jumped on the subway, Noanie and Pop included. Ava and Wyatt had to be dropped off at the upper school in Gramercy, and afterward we took Anna down to her school a few blocks south. The 6 train was a lifesaver on these busy mornings.

The big event for the little ones, from kindergarten through third grade, is an adorable Halloween march through the city. The children, who have all transformed into superheroes and princesses, zombies and witches, march around the block with their parents to a police station, where officers hand out candy.

Once again, I was amazed by how festive everything felt. On a typical workday, Andrew would have been Dad on Duty, and I would have shown up (after madly tearing down Park Avenue from Times Square) to make it for the last fifteen minutes of the parade, so I was truly thankful to be there. I talked to other parents, complimented all the kids' costumes, and pretended that everything was normal. No one observing our happy little family unit had any idea what was actually going through our minds.

After the parade, with the kids hopped up on candy and back at their desks, my parents, Andrew, and I went to a little diner nearby for breakfast. We were wired with anxiety and couldn't eat much, so we mostly drank coffee and continued to talk about what was next.

"You're really going to like Dr. Axelrod," I told my family. "But she was pushing me toward a lumpectomy. She seemed a bit taken aback when I mentioned mastectomy. Then again, I'm not even sure how much I remember from our meeting. I was pretty out of it yesterday."

"Well, it's good that we can all be there this morning to hear what she has to say. We can go from there," said my dad.

With so many decisions ahead of us, we all mentioned how grateful we were to have my brother, the doctor, for guidance. In less than an hour, we would have the results of the MRI, and those would give us a much clearer picture of exactly what we were facing over the months and years to come.

Just before ten, we were back at the glass-and-steel NYU building with the word "cancer" looming over the doorway. As we filed in to meet with Dr. Axelrod, I spotted a familiar face. It was Russ Marhull, the photographer who'd taped my announcement about my on-air mammogram.

Our eyes met. I gave him a hug and said, "What are you doing here?"

He said, "Why are *you* here?" Then we both teared up. "My ex-wife. She just got diagnosed. Please tell me that's not why you're here."

"It is," I said.

"Oh, my God, this is unbelievable."

Russ and I hugged again, and it seemed like some bad cosmic joke—the two of us, on the same day, at the same time, in the same surgeon's office. But then he explained how her diagnosis came about. After working on the "Go Pink" broadcast, he'd urged her to get a mammogram, and sure enough, her results were positive.

My parents, Andrew, and I were shown to the same small office with the love seat and the coffee table where I'd sat in stunned tears yesterday. It was a tight space for four people. I glanced at the photos on the desk and bulletin board and saw glimpses of Dr. Axelrod the person, not just the surgeon. There she was posing with her son, her friends, her husband. On the wall, there was even a framed cover of a breast cancer book she wrote with Rosie O'Donnell called *Bosom Buddies: Lessons and Laughter on Breast Health and Cancer* (*If she's Rosie's doctor, then I must be in good hands,* I thought). I hadn't noticed any of those details in the blur of the day before.

A moment later, Dr. Axelrod came in, wearing a lab coat over a light wool suit, and we faced the moment of truth.

"Let's look at the MRI," she said. She pulled up the images on her computer and used a pen to point out the tumor. "It's just under two centimeters," she said. "But my biggest concern is that, given where it's located, you may lose your nipple." Then she pulled up some images of nipple tattoos. "I want to get you accustomed to the thought of it," she said. "I know it takes a while to absorb all of this."

She talked about my surgical options—lumpectomy, mastectomy, or bilateral mastectomy and reconstruction—and she kept emphasizing how it was all going to look, which didn't really resonate with me.

I'd already told her, "I don't care how it looks." The fact is, I didn't care about whether or not I had to have a tattoo instead of a nipple. I didn't care about reconstruction. At the moment, all the cosmetic issues seemed superficial and silly. All I cared about was living, about getting through this, about getting the cancer OUT.

"Trust me, Amy," she said. "You will care. You're a forty-year-old woman. This stuff is important. A year or two down the road you're going to wish you'd put more thought into the process."

She came back to my surgical options and began to talk about the lumpectomy. After a moment, I couldn't listen anymore, and I said, even more resolutely than I had the day before, "I want a bilateral mastectomy."

She waited a beat, glancing at each of us in turn. Then she said, "Okay, I'll support that. It's your decision."

My parents looked at each other, and my mother had tears in her eyes. But the fact is, if they'd said I had to cut my arm off, I'd have had them do it right then and there. I was totally committed to whatever I needed to do to give me my best shot with the least amount of worry and concern afterward.

Dr. Axelrod continued in her reassuringly no-nonsense way. "I have a preferred plastic surgeon, Dr. Mihye Choi, to do the reconstruction, so she'll be in the operating room with me for the first procedure. I want you to meet with her, and I want her to tell you exactly what you're going to be in for from beginning to end. This will require a huge investment of time on your part. There are a number of surgeries involved, and it's uncomfortable."

I swallowed hard, but I wasn't choosing this course of action because I thought it was the *easy* way out.

"It's a very grueling and long surgery," she continued. "You'll have drains in you for weeks, and they'll have to be cleaned and changed every couple of hours. It's also a long recovery—up to six weeks—and most often with physical therapy afterward. Also, you'll have no feeling in your chest for at least two years." She did another survey of our faces, the four of us staring back at her, hanging on her every word. "Sometimes the sensation comes back," she continued, "but it probably won't. You may never feel anything in your nipples, which is no small thing. It's something you can't really prepare for, but you need to know."

None of this was pleasant to hear. In fact, it didn't seem real—*how the hell, in the course of twenty-four hours, did I go from a follow-up mammogram to nipple tattoos?*—but it didn't shake my conviction that bilateral mastectomy was the right choice. I was so focused on that that I pushed away all thoughts about what I would look like or feel like after surgery. I was, however, struck by how odd it was that the patient, rather than the surgeon, decided which procedure to have. If my brother hadn't advised me, I'm pretty sure I would have gone with the lumpectomy, which Dr. Axelrod had been steering me toward. She never made an outright recommendation, but she was definitely saying, *Hey, this is a much easier surgery, and it looks like your tumor is isolated, so why go through something grueling if you don't have to?*

But there was still so much the doctors didn't know. Had it spread to my lymph nodes? Had it spread anywhere else? No one was going to tell me what I had to do, and yet deep down I knew. I wanted to avoid years of monitoring and give myself the best opportunity for fewer procedures down the road. I was thinking about my children, because of course I wanted to provide for them and see them grow and flourish and have children of their own. I loved life. I loved my job. I loved living in New York City. I wasn't ready to let anything stop me, or even slow me down. Actually, when I thought about this disease threatening the wonderful life I'd built with Andrew, it made me mad. It made me want to fight back.

Dr. Axelrod went on to explain how during the surgery they would take out the sentinel lymph node to see if the cancer had spread. If it had, they'd have to take out more. She prepared me for just how painful this would be, because they'd have to cut through the muscle under my arm. She also said that the day before surgery I would have radioactive dye injected underneath my arm to "light up" the lymph nodes so the surgeons could find them.

"There's a lot we don't know," she said. "We won't even know the stage of your cancer until we get in there. But we'll have pathology standing by. We'll get the tumor out. We'll look at the lymph nodes, and then we'll know a lot more."

The ball was rolling. I had my plan. I was going to be aggressive, and as we stood to leave, I felt the momentum and power of knowing what I was going to do next. Dr. Axelrod had arranged for us to see the plastic surgeon, Dr. Choi, right away, and we headed to her office just thirteen blocks away. It was beautiful and Zen-like, appointed with orchids and white marble, very modern and spacious. Even though she was in private practice, she'd agreed to take the standard fee of an NYU staff plastic surgeon for my procedure. Getting her on my team was huge, because she did reconstructive breast surgery every single week.

The nurse had me undress and stand in front of a camera. She took a number of pictures, because, as she explained it, Dr. Choi would try to make my final outcome resemble what I'd looked like before. *This is the last documentation of the young, healthy me,* I thought. It was like taking pictures of a building before tearing it down. As the nurse worked, Dr. Choi explained the concept of expanders, which are kind of like those Capri Sun juice pouches that kids drink. She would insert the devices to temporarily replace my breast tissue and prevent my skin from contracting, so it would be pliant and ready for reconstruction. The jury was still out on whether or not I would need chemo—I was hopeful that I could avoid it—but if I did, I would have to wait until the treatment was over before having the reconstructive second surgery. So we had to plan for every eventuality, because each decision affected the next.

Dr. Choi was very kind and reassuring, telling me that I was going to look beautiful and that I was going to be okay. But this had been an incredible amount of detail to absorb, all of it fraught with emotion, so by the time we got back to our apartment, I was exhausted. And tonight was Halloween—in just a little while we would pick up the kids and head out to trick-or-treat.

I had only about an hour to rest, but there was no way I could slow my thoughts down enough to relax, let alone nap. I was pacing the apartment when my mom made a suggestion: "Would it help if you called someone who knows exactly what you're going through right now? Someone like Robin or Hoda?"

I immediately perked up. Hoda Kotb is the co-anchor for the fourth hour of *Today;* she and I had shared a dressing room for almost a year when I was at NBC and had grown very close. We'd gone through divorces within a year of each other, and though she never talked about it much, she was a breast cancer survivor.

But first I called Robin. She was the one who'd convinced me to have that mammogram, and so I had to thank her for potentially saving my life. I sent her an email and asked her to call me as soon as she had a free moment. My phone rang almost immediately.

"Hey, Amy, what's up?"

Sitting on my bed, door closed, I said, "I don't know how to say this to you, but I need to let you know I had a follow-up mammogram yesterday, and I found out . . . I have breast cancer." I began to cry.

"Oh, my gosh. Oh, my gosh, Amy. I am shocked. I cannot believe this." But then she shifted gears and said, "Let me just tell you this right now. You're going to be okay."

I told her the few details I knew about my diagnosis so far and that I wanted to know about her own experience. I asked her about her stage at the time of diagnosis, her surgery, her doctors, and any advice she had for me. I desperately wanted to hear someone else's story and the choices they made. Robin was very frank with me and incredibly supportive. One of the things she told me was: "Keep your mind open. Keep your options open. Get as much information as you can, and know that the information is going to change."

I nodded as she spoke, taking it all in from the voice of hard-won experience.

"What doctors think they know now may not end up being the reality," she added. "You get this diagnosis. You want to have all the information, but it's going to change. Medicine is not an exact science, and they only know what they know *today*. There will be surprises along the way." Then she confirmed what I'd been feeling and the way I'd approached things so far. "Amy," she said, "everyone's cancer is different. Don't let anyone tell you what you have to do. You have to do what you feel is right."

I felt so much better. Speaking to Robin reminded me of my power as a patient.

Next I called Hoda, and she answered right away. It had been about a year since we'd spoken on the phone, when she called to congratulate me on my new position at ABC. With Hoda, you pick up right where you left off, and so she started with an enthusiastic "Amy! How are you, friend?"

"Not so great," I said. I launched in about my diagnosis. Hoda echoed Robin's shock and sadness, but within a few seconds she jumped ahead to "What can I do? I'm coming over. I'm going to bring you a care package of my favorite things. I'm going to take care of you."

I was so happy I'd made the call. My friend, whom I missed seeing every day, was now making me feel so much better. Just like Robin, she was extremely open about her own experience with breast cancer. Then she added an anecdote that made all the difference. When she was first diagnosed, she was working on *Dateline,* so she had to tell her boss and producer, David Corvo. As she told it, he said to her, "Hoda, I know a lot of breast cancer survivors, and they all have one thing in common."

"What's that?"

"They're still alive."

I know that people die of breast cancer every day and that others survive for years. But in those early days after diagnosis, you feel like it's an immediate death sentence. You can't escape the feeling of *I don't have much time left. I'm dying.* So hearing that little bit of encouragement was really powerful.

When I walked out of my bedroom, my mom asked, "Are you glad you called?"

"Definitely," I said. The weight of the world had fallen off me. Robin and Hoda had suffered through breast cancer, too, and emerged on the other end happy, successful, and energetic. They were *alive.* It meant everything to know I could call on them and ask them anything.

My hour was up, so we picked up the kids from school and stopped at home for necessary costume adjustments: Annalise was still a princess, Ava was an owl, and Wyatt was a ninja. Then all seven of us piled into our SUV to head up toward our house in Putnam County. The kids' Catholic school was out on Friday, November 1, for All Saints' Day, so our weekend had begun.

Our first stop was Bronxville, which is a beautiful town filled with gorgeous Tudor houses, tree-lined streets, and wide sidewalks for little trick-or-treaters. The neighborhood goes all out on holiday decorations—it's truly a perfect Halloween spot.

We took the kids by Tim's place first so he could see them dressed up and so the girls could see their little half sister, Carson, in her costume. My ex and I are on great terms, and while I usually give his wife, Jessica, a hug when I see her, this was one of the first times that Tim and I hugged since the divorce. I knew I'd remember the poignancy of that moment forever.

"I'm so sorry," he said.

Then he and Andrew shook hands, and I felt truly lucky. My parents, who have known Tim since he was nineteen years old, were giving hugs all around. In the face of devastation, I was so glad to know that my family could walk into my ex-husband's house with his new family, and everybody would be nothing but supportive and loving. Andrew, Ava, Anna, Wyatt, and I had all visited Jessica in the hospital the day after she gave birth to Carson. We sit together at class plays and ceremonies (Carson often wants to sit in *my* lap), and in those moments I look around and see so much beauty. I'm incredibly proud of how we've all worked hard to create a cohesive and loving, if unconventional, family for our children.

"If there's anything we can do," Tim said, "we'll do it."

Standing in the doorway, little Carson said, "Can I come with you, Miss Amy?" I covered her with kisses and told her we'd see her soon.

It was a foggy, very Halloween-y night, and we followed the kids as they made their rounds, the parents and grandparents hanging back with our flashlights as our little goblins ran up to each house. Everything seemed so perfect—and yet I had been fielding calls all afternoon and evening as more and more colleagues heard my news. Barbara Fedida was thoughtfully checking in every few hours to make sure I had everything I needed, and Ben Sherwood called to see if there was anything he could do to help. Dr. Jen Ashton, who had been there during my on-air mammogram, called to see if she could provide any medical support. It felt bizarre to straddle my two realities—dealing with an unfolding medical tragedy and watching an excited trio of children enjoy the best life could offer them in that moment: fantasy, candy, and chocolate. It began to rain, so we piled into our car, the kids in the back, giggling and singing as we headed north out of West-chester.

The kids were swapping candy as we made our way through the misty fog on U.S. Route 9, a two-lane road that twists and turns along the banks of the Hudson River. But despite the delicious sound of their sugar-induced laughter, my mood suddenly darkened. My throat tightened, my heart palpitated, and my breathing became shallow and quick. I felt as if I couldn't swallow and started gasping for air. I tried to breathe through my nose, roll down the window—anything to feel like I wasn't going to choke. Unable to get air to my lungs, I cried to Andrew, "Pull the car over now. I have to get out of this car. RIGHT. NOW." By then we were in a torrential downpour, and I didn't care. I would open the door and jump out if I had to.

Andrew pulled over, and he and my dad held me as I stood there, gasping for air, hyperventilating and sobbing. It was a full-on panic attack like I had never experienced before, and it was happening on the side of a dark rainy road on Halloween—how's that for scary?

My dad went back into the car to tell the kids I just felt a little sick. Andrew kept holding me and telling me it was going to be all right. The problem was, I knew that wasn't true. Nothing was going to be okay again. Nothing would ever be the same. Would I always be this scared? How hard was it going to be to put on this "normal" life for my kids while on the inside I felt as if everything was falling apart and out of my control? I didn't say any of this out loud. Instead, soaking wet, I finally got back into the car and finished the trip with my head sticking out the window, not caring that the cold wind was hitting my even colder, wetter face.

The next day, Dr. Axelrod prescribed Ativan for my anxiety—the first of many medications that would (depressingly) begin to fill my medicine cabinet.

Chapter Three

"I Have Breast Cancer"

That weekend upstate was filled with calls, texts, and emails from close colleagues, and the news spread, as these things do; over the next two weeks, enough bouquets arrived for me to open a floral shop. All the same, it was wrenching to repeat the story to each and every well-intentioned friend who called. I felt a tremendous urge to just get it all out in the open. I wanted to be free of the information almost as much as I wanted to be liberated from the cancer itself.

I spent a lot of time FaceTiming with my brother that weekend in the country, going over all of my options, and I felt more determined than ever to go forward with my initial gut decision: a double mastectomy. Saturday afternoon, we hiked around the wildlife preserve that borders our property. My parents, Andrew, and I all climbed to the top of a rock from which we could see the Hudson River against the fall colors, the oranges and reds and yellows glowing as if the hillside were ablaze. We brought a bottle of champagne and some plastic cups and toasted to the future as the sun set. I took it all in, still absorbing the shock of everything that had happened in just a couple of days, and feeling very lucky to be alive.

On Sunday afternoon we had to go back to the city, because the kids had school on Monday and I had a slew of doctors' appointments, including a trip to the pediatrician with the kids to get their flu shots. That week I was supposed to fly to Miami, to fill in as host of Jorge Ramos's show on Fusion TV, our Hispanic channel. Instead, I lay low, only venturing out to meet with doctors for pre-op visits.

That week I received a welcome surprise. Hoda showed up at my apartment with a huge basket filled with all her favorite beauty products. She laughed and said she'd been stalking me. We didn't have a doorman, so she had stopped by a few times but couldn't get in, and she kept coming back until we were home. I still have the shampoo and conditioner she gave me. It's funny how powerful a sensory memory can be. Every time I smell them, I feel her love.

I was headed toward major surgery, and there were still so many unanswered questions. The one thing I did know was that Dr. Smith was right—having that mammogram had given me the best chance at survival.

I'd taken the time now to absorb my new reality, and I finally felt like I was ready to face my colleagues (and the cameras) before my operation. A part of me just wanted to say the words out loud and be done with it: "I have breast cancer." I've always believed there is something cathartic about owning the worst possible truth. Keeping it a secret gives it power, but acknowledging it sets you free. I talked with Tom Cibrowski, the then-EP of *Good Morning America,* and told him I wanted to go on air with my diagnosis, before my surgery. With my double mastectomy scheduled for Thursday, November 14, we agreed the best time for my announcement would be on Monday, November 11.

I SNEAKED INTO ABC headquarters in jeans and a sweatshirt later that week to meet with producer Thea Trachtenberg. Tom had privately told her about my breast cancer and asked her to work with me on the piece. She was so kind and shared with me some of her own health struggles, to let me know I wasn't alone. It was incredible how connected I felt to anyone else who had walked a similar path. We discussed what I was willing to share in the piece and what I wasn't (like the sonogram image of my tumor). I gave her my doctors' names and numbers, as Thea wanted to completely understand my medical situation before putting all the elements together. I knew my story was in good hands.

Then I had to run down to the third-floor audio booth to track my voice for a story that was set to air that night, on country-music megastar Luke Bryan. He had opened up to me about the tragic and sudden loss of both of his siblings in separate accidents, something he had never before talked about publicly. I had done the emotional interview in Nashville just a few weeks earlier. Now I got so upset in the tracking booth that I had to stop several times to collect myself. Everything was so raw. Even speaking about someone else's death choked me up. My *20/20* producers had no idea what was going on with my health, and I'm sure they were a bit confused. "I'm sorry, guys, give me a second," I had to say a few times. I knew they would put two and two together when they heard my announcement the following week. I also knew in that moment that going back to work was going to be difficult and that Monday would test my strength.

That evening, my family sat down to watch the Luke Bryan piece, which was airing as part of the special *In the Spotlight with Robin Roberts.* When the interview popped up on the TV, I shuddered. It was chilling to watch my carefree self—the person I was only a few *weeks* ago—wearing jeans and a smile and walking around Luke's catfish pond. I looked so healthy and so *innocent,* with no idea of what was waiting for me just around the bend. Then I experienced another eerie, prescient moment, which gave me goose bumps.

"You've been very private about this side of your life. Why is it important for you to talk about it now?" I asked him.

"My main thing is, it's important for people to know they're not alone," Luke said. "I love the fact that people can see that God still is gracious and, and humbling and powerful and can make things right, too. And if me telling my story moves people down a positive path of hope and getting up out of bed and getting that going, then, you know, it's certainly worth telling."

That exchange was like a message in a bottle I'd written to myself to find only a few weeks later. It was as if Luke were speaking to me, not down in Georgia in mid-October, but on this Tuesday night in New York City. His words of encouragement soon became mine. I was certain that once I shared my story, other people would walk with me, and I with them.

I DIDN'T TELL my grandmother until that Sunday, the day before going public. I knew she was going to take the news extremely hard, so I wanted to give her every moment I could of blissful innocence. She and my grandfather were both in poor health, and I worried about adding any unnecessary stress, but I knew she was an avid watcher of *Good Morning America,* and I had to tell her first. My grandmother is a tough Southern lady who grew up along the Mississippi coast, worked hard her entire life, and gave birth to ten children. When I was in high school, she always encouraged me to get in front of the camera and onstage. She would sign me up for auditions she'd read about in the paper—without asking me first—and then make sure I went. When I was older, my mom told me that my grandmother had always dreamed of becoming a journalist but instead poured herself into her children and ultimately her grandchildren (and great-grandchildren).

Thankfully, three of my mom's sisters live in the Atlanta area, five minutes from my grandmother's house, and all three of them—Aunts Kathy, Patty, and Leslie—volunteered to break the news face-to-face. Mom and I set up a time to call while my aunts were still by her side.

She cried, and I tried to reassure her, but it was tough. In all her eighty-eight years, she'd never received a call like that one. And while it was incredibly sad for all of us, it was also an odd position to be in, and one I was getting familiar with: When you have cancer, you often end up consoling everyone else. You tell them, *I'm going to be all right.* You say, *I'm a fighter; I'm strong; I'll make it through this, don't worry.* You tell them that you'll survive, even if you don't believe it yourself.

Now that everyone who needed to hear my news directly from me had, it was time to tell the world. Riding in to work the next morning, I was nervous but relieved. I was also excited to see my friends and colleagues, but Dr. Axelrod had cautioned me about how I would likely be treated after making the big announcement on television. "Amy," she said, "I'm guessing you've never really been pitied before, and you need to prepare yourself for it. To be pitied can be a pretty awful thing. Make sure you've thought this through."

Her words lingered in my head when I walked into our studio in Times Square for the first time in two weeks. It was strange: My world had become this dark, surreal landscape, and yet here was my workplace, bright and cheery and filled with smiling faces. As I was getting ready in my dressing room, each of my bosses came by to show their support: Barbara Fedida, Ben Sherwood, James Goldston (the current president of ABC News), as well as Tom Cibrowski and Jeffrey Schneider (then–senior VP of communications). They were loving, but no one really knew what to say. Their presence alone meant the world, but I felt overwhelmed. Dr. Axelrod was right: Even well-intentioned pity is difficult to absorb and accept. I've always been someone who loves to come in, keep my head down, and do good work—and then work some more. I'm not so keen on attention—it makes me feel awkward, and *this* kind of attention felt . . . well, excruciating.

Mom and Dad had decided that they were better off shielding my kids from my television appearance, so they stayed home to make sure the TV wasn't turned on before school. Andrew arrived at the studios around eight o'clock to support me, timing it just before I went on the air so he wouldn't distract me or add to the emotional scene.

When we'd planned my appearance, Thea, Kaitlyn, and I agreed it might be best to put the diagnosis in the piece. I didn't think I was emotionally strong enough to say the words "I have breast cancer" on live television, so I'd asked if I could simply track that statement—meaning that we would reveal it in the prerecorded piece. But as I was getting ready to go on, Tom Cibrowski came back into my dressing room and said, "Amy, I really think you need to give us your diagnosis leading into your spot. Otherwise, it's going to be a little bit confusing. If you're up for it, I think it's important for *you* to say, 'I have breast cancer,' and then we'll immediately cut to the piece." I understood and agreed to do it. Now I was getting really nervous.

At 8:15 A.M., I sat on the *GMA* couch between Robin Roberts and Dr. Jen Ashton, the two people who were with me just weeks earlier when I walked into that mammovan. We held hands as I made my announcement. I was determined not to cry, but pain and fear were written all over my face. What gave me courage was the impact of my message. I knew that the moment I told our viewers I had breast cancer, most women watching who were putting off their own mammogram appointments wouldn't wait any longer. I felt certain lives would be saved. This was real—and it was life or death. *GMA* had literally saved my life, and I wanted to pay it forward.

Robin began. "Our good friend Amy Robach is here. She has some very important news to share. Last month you may remember that she took a very brave step live here on *Good Morning America*, getting a mammogram. It was part of our pink initiative. Amy, the floor is yours."

I took a deep breath and squeezed their hands.

"Thank you very much, Robin," I said. "I decided to take one for the team. This was, for me, about public service, because you all know I didn't *really* want to have that mammogram. Well, just a few short weeks later, words I never expected to hear, I was told that I have breast cancer."

That was the roll cue for my recorded piece. The package was beautiful, beginning with my on-air mammogram and ending with pictures of my daughters and my family and me saying that I had a lot to fight for; it brought a few tears down my cheeks, which I quickly wiped away before the camera came back live to me.

"It is absolutely surreal to be sitting here," I said. "But as scary as it all is, I am so, so lucky because you guys pushed me into that mammovan, and thank God you did, because I know me, and I wasn't in any rush to have that done anytime soon."

Robin and Jen and I talked for several minutes about my options for treatment. Robin said, "These have been very difficult weeks for you. Can you just share what you've decided to do?"

"I have decided to have a bilateral mastectomy. And what comes next? We're not sure yet. I don't know about chemo; I don't know what stage I am; I don't know if it's spread. So we'll find out those things in the weeks to come. So this—this time is the hardest part, the limbo, when you don't know," I said.

But there was more I wanted to share. "And I'm saying this out loud because my whole, the whole reason why I walked into that van was to raise awareness for people to get mammograms, and little did I know that I would be a walking example of having a mammogram save my life. Robin, you pushed me to do this—YOU saved my life. ABC News saved my life."

"You saved your life, Amy, you did it," said Robin. She took my hand once again, and after offering warm words and reassurance, added, "Your husband's here." Andrew joined us on camera, along with George Stephanopoulos, Lara Spencer, and Josh Elliott. The segment ended with Andrew, all of my colleagues, and me in a circle of strength.

When we went to commercial break, I felt light and free. I let out a big sigh and an even bigger smile. "I'm really glad that's over," I said.

Robin turned and looked at me. She said, "Oh, it's not over. It's just beginning."

———

OF ALL PEOPLE, Robin knew *exactly* what was going to happen next. The response—from the media, from friends I hadn't spoken to in years, from colleagues I'd worked with decades earlier, and from complete strangers—was incredible and intense. That night, I was one of the lead stories on the local news and entertainment shows. Over on CNN, Piers Morgan spent the last half hour of his show discussing how my on-air mammogram had led to "Robach's Shocking Cancer Diagnosis." Those were the actual words on the bottom of the screen! I had spent my entire career telling other people's stories, and it was bizarre to *become* the story.

Early the next morning, I got a text from my old boss Don Nash, executive producer of *Today,* telling me to watch their show at 8:00 A.M. My former colleagues Matt Lauer, Savannah Guthrie, Natalie Morales, and Al Roker all wished me well, sending love from across town. It touched me immensely. My house filled up with flowers and cards.

After my surgery, Marly, my assistant, emailed me from our uptown offices and said, "You've got to pick all this up. And bring your car! Your office—you can't even walk in it. There are so many boxes and letters."

We drove over and waited while Marly rolled an overflowing mail cart down 66th Street so we could take it all home.

When we got back, I sat on the floor and opened every single letter and package. I had never felt so connected to so many people I'd never even met. Women from all over the country told me their stories and sent me their cancer pictures—images of them running in races and losing their hair, but all with big, beautiful smiles of strength. One Texas group sent a picture of thirty survivors, all dressed in pink and standing up to cheer me on, printed on a big blanket. It said: YOU'VE GOT THIS, AMY.

I wept as I saw how beautiful every one of these women was, inside and out. It restored any faith I had lost in the kindness of strangers and simply blew me away. People sent me robes and bras for double mastectomies and all kinds of gadgets I didn't know existed, like a supportive pillow that had a pocket for the TV remote. Women knitted me caps and hats for hair loss and blankets for chemo, because you get cold during treatment. Others put together care packages complete with mouth lozenges (because your mouth gets dry) and ginger for nausea. One woman told me I should wear lip gloss and high heels if I had to go to chemo. "Go in there and look amazing," she wrote. It's impossible to fully express my gratitude for the collective hug I felt from survivors all over this country. Each and every gesture of love and support gave me strength I didn't know I had.

ON WEDNESDAY, IT was time to hug and kiss my daughters goodbye. I couldn't spend my pre-surgery night with them, because the doctors had to "light up" my lymph nodes, which would make me radioactive and dangerous for them to be around. I knew they would visit me in the hospital the following day, but it was still torture to tear myself away.

Andrew and I went back to the NYU Cancer Center, where doctors lifted up my arm and injected me with the radioactive dye so Dr. Axelrod could find my lymph nodes during the double mastectomy and test them for cancer.

Perhaps just as painful, I went straight from the doctor's office to my attorney's office to draw up a will. I had never rewritten my original one after my divorce, and now, with new assets and a second marriage, I needed to get my affairs in order. At least, I felt like I needed to. I wanted to feel at peace before heading into the operating room. Staring down at those documents not only forced me to confront mortality; it also made me realize how little time Andrew and I had actually been together. I had to make decisions like: *How do I split up my 401(k)s, my savings, and my jewelry between my daughters and my husband? Who's going to be the proxy if I go into a coma?* Perhaps because we had been married for only three and a half years, we had never thought about any of this, and now I had to come to grips with: *Are you my next of kin, or is my mother?*

With Andrew by my side, we signed our wills and didn't say much at all. We both knew how much the other one was hurting.

We stayed that night at the Library Hotel on Madison Avenue, not far from NYU Medical Center. It was a beautiful room, but it seemed weird to be in a romantic hotel, away from our children, with the anxiety building by the minute. To take my mind off the surgery, my parents and Kaitlyn met us at Dos Caminos on Park and 27th, for Mexican food and margaritas. It sounds oddly festive, I know, but it's my favorite food, and I wanted the night to be as much fun as possible, for all of us. Who knew when we'd have another like it? Sitting at that table, laughing and drinking, we did our best to ignore the unspoken fear hanging over us.

We lingered as long as possible. I wanted to be good and tired, to try to turn off my brain and maybe even get some sleep that night. Eventually, Mom and Dad had to relieve our babysitter, but before saying goodbye, we decided that they would come to the hospital with me in the morning. Kaley would go to the apartment at five-thirty and get the girls to school.

We hugged goodbye and tried not to cry. "I love you guys. See you tomorrow," I said.

Andrew and I walked out into the crisp evening air, back to our hotel room. I was so scared. He held me in bed as I wiped away more tears.

"I promise you, you're going to do fine," he said. "We are all going to be by your side every step of the way. You're in good hands, baby." And I did fall asleep quickly, thanks to an Ativan from Dr. Axelrod.

The next morning, my parents were waiting for us downstairs in the car, and we were all bursting with nerves as we made the quick trip over to First Avenue.

"How are you feeling, honey?" asked my mom.

"As good as can be expected, I guess." I actually thought I might throw up.

"You're going to do great, sweetheart," said my dad.

Andrew squeezed my hand and gave me a kiss.

It was just past six-fifteen when we arrived at NYU. Eight years earlier, I'd walked through those very same doors on the morning I gave birth to my little Annalise. I remembered the security guard who'd asked me if I was having twins as I made my way to the maternity wing.

"No," I said, "there's just one in there."

"Are you sure?" he asked.

This time there was no mouthy guard at the entrance, only Andrew, my parents, and me, anxiously heading to the tenth floor for surgery.

I tried to remain calm, but all I could think was, *Please God, please God, don't let it have spread,* on an endless loop.

Dr. Axelrod had told me to bring my iPod and earphones to the hospital. "I want you to be in a good place when we put you under. You should be listening to something you love, so pick out your favorite song," she'd said.

My parents waited outside the pre-op room. Andrew stayed with me as I changed into my hospital gown and the nurse inserted the IV. Finally, it was time. The nurse brought in a wheelchair.

"Do I have to ride in that down to the operating room?" I asked. I wanted to feel strong. I needed to feel my legs beneath me and to be in control one last time that day. I hugged Andrew and tried to sound brave.

"I'll see you soon," I said. "I love you."

"I love you, too."

And so I walked out of the room and down that hall, with an IV machine on one side of me and a nurse on the other. I turned around just as I was about to go through the OR doors and saw my parents and Andrew all standing together with big smiles, waving at me. I waved back and gave them all a thumbs-up.

The doors swung shut and my bravado evaporated. As the nurses helped me up onto the operating table and strapped down my arms and legs, I also became paralyzed with fear. I started crying, at first softly—trying desperately to control the tears—and eventually pretty hard, making noises and gulping. The nurses did everything they could to comfort me, making jokes, giving me warm blankets. They even turned on a heating pad under the sheet.

Dr. Axelrod and Dr. Choi came in, and they were both smiling and kind, but it was pretty obvious I was in distress. My mind was racing. I worried about everything from not waking up at all to what the news would be when I did. *What are they going to find? Has my cancer spread? What will I look like after losing my breasts? What will I feel like?*

It was Dr. Choi's job to put in the expanders to ready my body for reconstructive surgery later. Dr. Axelrod's was to make sure all the cancerous tissue was removed.

She asked me, "Do you have your song?"

I said, "Yes."

"Well, why don't you go ahead and start playing it."

I pressed PLAY, but with the IV dripping and the mask over my face, I probably heard only about thirty seconds. I'd chosen The Band Perry's "Pioneer." The words were perfect:

Oh, pioneer
I sing your song
It's the hymn of those who've gone before and those who carry
on. . . .

That's about all I heard, and then I woke up . . . in excruciating pain.

Some people say crazy things when they first come out of anesthesia, and maybe I did, too. But the first thing I *remember* saying when I woke up in the recovery room was, "Did it spread to my lymph nodes?"

Andrew was sitting beside me, holding my hand, and I was still out of it, but I kept asking him, "Is it in my lymph nodes? Is it in my lymph nodes?"

"Yes," he said. "But just your sentinel node."

He was brushing the hair out of my face and doing his best to look positive, but this was devastating news, and I could see it in his eyes.

I was already in more pain than I'd ever felt, and now I simply lost it and began to cry—and it *hurt* to cry! I could barely breathe through the pressure and throbbing in my chest and arms. I was nauseated and emotionally drained.

Apparently, when Dr. Axelrod came out of the OR to break the news to my family, Andrew had asked, "Who should tell her?"

Dr. Axelrod had said she wanted to explain it all to me but added, "She's going to have a pretty good idea when she wakes up, because of the significant pain under her arm." She had told me before the surgery that if they checked the sentinel node and it wasn't malignant, she wouldn't have to take any more out, and it wouldn't be too uncomfortable. If the cancer was in the sentinel node, they would have to go in deep, under the arm, and cut through tissue, which is extremely painful. No doubt, the pain under my arm was unbearable, but so was the pain in my chest, and coming out of anesthesia, my head was not exactly primed and ready for putting two and two together. Dr. Axelrod ended up removing thirteen lymph nodes. And she had more news for me in that recovery room.

I was miserable, but she had a big smile on her face. "You were good, Amy," she said. "You had a gut feeling from the beginning about having the mastectomy, and it turns out there was reason for it. So you were good, but I was good, too. I found a second tumor that we wouldn't have found if we'd just done the lumpectomy."

I started crying again. I don't know if it was from gratitude that she had caught it or terror that there was more cancer than we'd thought.

"I made one last sweep with my index finger of your chest cavity," she said, "and I felt a bump. So I took a little piece of it and sent it to pathology. It was smaller than the first tumor, but sure enough it was malignant."

Upon further testing of all the tissue they removed, the pathologist found that my breast had a number of pre-cancerous cells, as well. Turns out, I was the poster child for mastectomy, but no one knew it ahead of time, because my lymph nodes "looked" normal in the sonogram and my tumor seemed to be isolated.

After a while, I realized there was another doctor next to Dr. Axelrod: my ob-gyn, Dr. Ilene Fischer.

"I wanted to be here when you woke up," she said, "and to tell you how terrible I feel that you were alone when you got your diagnosis. I made it seem as if the follow-up images were nothing to be alarmed about. I feel like I was the reason you were alone on that day, and I'm sorry." Her desire to support me at that moment was sweet and moving, but I couldn't blame her for how my diagnosis played out. No one had seen this coming.

It was early afternoon at this point, and I was fighting tremendous nausea. The nurses gave me meds to try to stop me from throwing up, but nothing worked. At a certain point, they couldn't give me any more drugs through my IV. "We can give you something," they said, "but it's a very painful injection."

"Fine," I said. "I don't care. I'll do anything to make this nausea go away."

As predicted, I moaned and jerked as the nurse injected me in my thigh—later, there was a raised, bruised area where the needle went in, which makes me think she must have hit a nerve. But the insult added to injury was that it didn't work. I had never felt so sick.

Dr. Choi had suggested that we hire a private nurse for that first night. The care at NYU is excellent, but it's such a busy place that they can't tend to you minute by minute when your needs are really intense. After a surgery like this, mine were. By five o'clock I was in my own room with the nurse. Andrew and my parents were there, and Kaitlyn had picked the kids up from school and—with my blessing—loaded them up with all the things I usually won't let them eat. But they really wanted to come see me, so at around seven she brought them to the hospital.

My memory is blurry because I was in so much pain, but I do re-member seeing fear on my daughters' faces as they looked at me. An-nalise was crying. In hindsight, it probably wasn't a good idea to see them, because I was in a horrific place, and it showed. The girls brought me drawings, and Ava crawled into the bed with me and put her head next to mine on the pillow, saying, "Mommy, I love you. You're going to be okay. I promise."

I couldn't believe how strong my ten-year-old was.

That night Andrew slept in a chair next to me on one side, with the nurse on the other. She ended up being a godsend, because the pain was awful, and the nausea was only getting worse. I kept moaning and could barely move. Finally the nurse said, "You have to get up and walk. It's the only way you're going to get that anesthesia out of you."

"I can't walk," I told her, incredulous. "I can't even sit up right now."

"Yes, you can. And, with my help, you will." She explained that when you get up and move, your blood pressure and heart rate in-crease, which moves everything along and out of your system. She was an older Eastern European woman—with very strong arms; clearly, she'd done this before—and although it took about ten minutes of careful maneuvering, she got me off that bed.

I think I managed about three steps before I said, "I'm going to throw up," so Andrew grabbed the bedpan and I started retching. The IV fluids and lingering anesthesia all came up, burning my throat.

I got back in bed, but the nurse made me get up every couple of hours through the night, and each time she made me walk farther. She told me she was going to keep it up until I could walk the whole hall-way loop. She held one arm and Andrew held the other, and with my IV roller next to me, I shuffled down the corridor. At first I could barely move, and it was shocking how little control I had over my body. I'd been a gymnast, and I'm an avid runner, so it was extremely humbling—and frustrating. I'd only make it halfway before getting sick again and having to turn back. But she was a remarkable woman, a combination of loving mother and drill sergeant, and she just kept at it, until eventually . . . I did it. I never imagined I'd be so proud to walk a thousand feet without collapsing.

She told me she'd taken care of her mom when she died of breast cancer, and it became her mission to help women who were recovering from this kind of surgery. It was not a pleasant job, but even in my addled mental state, I felt inspired by her passion to help others.

A bilateral mastectomy usually requires a minimum of two nights in the hospital (they told me one night per breast), but I really wanted to get out of there in one. That was my main incentive to get up and walk. Every time I stood up, I felt like I was going to faint, but eventually the drugs cleared my system, and I started to feel *slightly* better.

When Dr. Axelrod came to visit me the next morning, she told me that maybe I could go home by the end of the day, which was just what I wanted to hear. Then she said, "Amy, I know you like to stay busy, but for the next several weeks you absolutely cannot lift anything. You're going to start to feel your strength coming back, but you have to take it slow. Even two weeks from now, on Thanksgiving, you can baste the turkey, but don't lift it." That made me smile. I laughed and promised to do nothing.

I left the hospital with three drains that had to be cleaned every couple of hours. I was in terrible shape, and all I wanted was a quiet evening at home—even if it was a quiet evening of pain pills, nausea, and fatigue. The girls were with their dad in Bronxville and Wyatt was with his mom, so it was just my parents, Andrew, and me.

But no sooner did we get home than one of my drains stopped working. I had one coming out of my armpit, where the lymph nodes had been removed, and one coming out of each breast, where I now had expanders inserted. The drain had been acting up while I was at the hospital, and the nurse had told me to keep a close eye on it. They prevent infection, so if one backs up, you're in trouble. My mom got really nervous. "We need to go back to the hospital," she said.

But the last thing I wanted to do was to go back to the hospital.

And as luck would have it, I didn't have to, because at around seven o'clock, as we were debating what to do, my brother, Eric, showed up at our front door. I was totally surprised and moved that he'd flown in, leaving his wife, three sons, and a very busy medical practice back in Georgia. Eric and I were extremely close when we were small, and then as we got into high school we became competitive in a nerdy kind of way, one-upping each other at SAT scores and GPAs. But we always complemented each other, because we're very different. I'm happy to be in front of any camera or microphone that comes my way, but my brilliant brother has always been shy. Once, he was being honored with a very prestigious medical award, and he was so embarrassed that he kept his head down and walked right into one of the monitors onstage. He's always been my guru for medical advice, and it was a huge relief to know that in this most vulnerable moment I had him watching over me.

He had barely put his bags down when Mom called him over to the couch to take a look at my malfunctioning drain. After a quick exam, he said, "Get me a steak knife and some glue." Dr. MacGyver to the rescue!

He opened up the tube and reinserted it properly, solving my first medical problem of the night in a matter of minutes. I was grateful beyond words. After that, Eric and Andrew took turns cleaning and changing my drains several times a day. Thanks to Eric, they were all working effectively.

I was happy to be home. I stayed on the couch the rest of that first night. Eric and I both love scary movies and convinced everyone else to watch *The Conjuring*. (Andrew and my parents can't stand scary movies, so this was a big give.) The movie was amazing and completely took my mind off the pain. The demon in that movie stops all the clocks at 3:07, so that weekend as I was recovering, we set the big clock in my kitchen to 3:07 and took the battery out. It's still that way, and every time I notice it, I laugh out loud.

I couldn't think of another time since my brother and I lived together that I had both Eric and my parents to myself. I felt safe, even while watching an evil spirit haunt a nice Rhode Island family. That night, with the kids away, Eric slept in the room with the bunk beds, and the next day, a Saturday, we piled into our SUV once again to go up to Putnam County, where we'd have more space. The car is big enough that I could lie flat across one of the seats, and Andrew drove as if he were transporting trays of glassware balanced on the roof. Leaving the immediate vicinity of my doctors was not the most prudent decision, and they had specifically told me not to get in a car, but my family agreed to the trip because my brother was with me (there's nothing quite like having a doctor in the family in moments like these). I needed to get as far away as I could—within reason—from hospitals and exam rooms. I can't imagine living anywhere other than New York, but I also love being in the middle of nowhere. We have a dirt driveway that's a quarter mile long, and as soon as I hear our wheels hit that gravel, my pulse slows and I know I'm home.

Eric had never been to our house and I was very excited for him to see it, but he'd missed all the beautiful fall colors. Now, only a few weeks after the Halloween weekend when we'd climbed the hill, the trees were nearly bare and the rocky outcrops exposed. The landscape looked bleak, harsh, and wintry. The house, though, a post-and-beam home built in the eighties, was still cozy. We lit a fire; I took up my position on the couch, and everybody circled around. I was still on a heavy regimen of pills that kept me foggy, but I felt comforted just hearing their voices around me as I drifted in and out.

Luckily for my family, there was some excitement on television that weekend: Georgia versus Auburn. Eric and I both went to UGA and are huge devotees. It was one of the best football games I've ever watched, with one of the worst endings for Georgia fans. We cheered and screamed through it all, especially after one of the most spectacular, victory-clenching Hail Mary passes of all time.

Before my surgery, my very good friend Sara Haines had bought me two special bras that accommodated drains, because if the drains swing or move, it *really* hurts. So I had on one of those, under a button-down shirt. Right before my surgery, Mom and I raced around Manhattan, looking for shirts with buttons—not something I usually wore—because I knew it would be weeks before I could lift my arms enough for a pullover. I was in a sad state, barely able to dress myself, unable to take a shower, so thank God my mother was there to help every step of the way. Mom was always at her finest form when we were sick as children, and she turned into SuperMom once again for me.

On Sunday afternoon, Eric had to get back to Georgia, his family, and his practice—and we had to get back to the city. We drove through Bronxville to pick up the kids at Tim's. They had school the next day, and I had a week filled with doctors' appointments.

BUT THE NEXT Friday, November 22, we decided to head back upstate and this time stay awhile. ABC told me to take as much time as I needed to recover, so that's exactly what I did. We asked the kids' teachers for their assignments and homeschooled them through Thanksgiving. My mom was a high school English teacher for most of her career, and she held daily lessons while I rested. I loved seeing my little girls and Wyatt at work around our dining table.

Before long, though, I got restless. I'm a doer, and I cannot stand just being. I'm no good at taking naps, or getting enough sleep, or relaxing in general. So, much to the chagrin of my mom, and despite my compromised physical condition, I decided to start taking on projects around the house. My parents drove me to Home Depot, where I picked out paints for our downstairs bedroom and my daughters' room. They watched helplessly as I slowly made my way up and down the aisles, grabbing supplies for additional projects, like tin tiles for the ceiling of our bathroom. I'm sure I looked crazy, with drains popping out at every angle and fatigue all over my face, stuffing home-improvement wares into my cart. But my parents were amazing: They knew they couldn't make me stop, so they helped me paint. My dad and Andrew installed those bathroom tiles, and I was thrilled that things were getting done. I was accomplishing *something*. The painting took me much longer than it normally would have, but the motion of that roller slowly going up and down was like physical therapy. The color of my daughters' bedroom was called Salt Pink, and it brightened up the room *and* my mood.

When I went to my post-surgical appointment with Dr. Axelrod a few weeks later, she couldn't believe my range of motion. She even called in a couple of nurses and had me show them how high I could lift my arms and how far back I could spread them. She had initially recommended a physical therapist but agreed that I didn't need it, because of my projects. After that, painting walls became part of my philosophy: Stay busy, move gracefully, and don't let anything stop you.

During those few weeks upstate, my children were on their best behavior, very kind and loving and sweet, and I saw the best come out in all of them. But these were also the days when my determination to stay upbeat and positive just abandoned me. Sometimes a wave of fear would spill over my body—when I was undressing, when I looked in the mirror, when I saw my scars. I had zero sensation in my chest, and whenever Andrew or the kids hugged me, it was a constant reminder of the trauma my body had gone through. I felt as if I had two hard foreign objects strapped to me that I had to carry around all day, and the mental weight of that was the hardest part. Sometimes I would crumble into the fetal position on my bed and cry. Andrew did everything he could do to help, but he was having a tough time of his own. He was still depressed over the death of his father five months before, and also dealing with a custody battle over Wyatt with his ex-wife, who'd moved to California after the divorce. So even while I was upstate, Andrew went back and forth to the city with Wyatt several times when his ex-wife came to visit.

Two weeks after my double mastectomy, it was time to meet with my oncologist, Dr. Ruth Oratz. It was the day before Thanksgiving, and I was nervous. But when we walked into her office, I noticed her photos—the Gobi Desert, treetops in the rain forest—and knew we would get along. A fellow adventurer and world traveler would probably relate to my need to keep moving even through cancer treatment, whatever that was going to be—and, boy, was I right. Dr. Oratz walked in with a kind smile, and I knew we were simpatico.

But despite our instant rapport, the news she had for me was not what I was hoping to hear. My doctors had sent my tumors and tissue to a lab in California, and Dr. Oratz had the pathology in a stack of papers in front of her. She recommended that I undergo chemotherapy, eight full rounds of a medium-strength concoction called CMF. Even though I'd tried to prepare myself, this was a tremendous blow. I listened as Dr. Oratz explained all the knowns and unknowns and how chemo reacted differently in everyone's body. I listened to side effects like bone aches and nausea and fatigue.

Her nurse, Beth, gave me pamphlets on hair loss and local wigmakers, as well as material on how your skin and body can react. Dr. Oratz wrote out about a dozen prescriptions, from anti-nauseants to anti-anxiety meds to steroids to injections—all things I would have to fill and have ready by December 16, just nine days before Christmas, the day of my first round of treatment.

It was so much to take in—how much my life had already changed, and how much it was about to change still. At least tomorrow was Thanksgiving, and I had so many things to be thankful for—namely, being alive.

BEFORE HEADING BACK upstate, I had a few errands to run, and Andrew had to tie up some loose ends at his office, so we split up and planned to meet back at Grand Central and take the train together at four o'clock. I actually had a hair appointment, of all things. After discussing my shoulder-length hair (and the fact that I might soon lose it) at the doctor's office, I decided to deal with my fear by joking with my longtime hairstylist, Laura, that she'd better do what she could with it now, before it was gone! We just trimmed it, and I thought I was handling everything pretty well. I was strong, I could deal with any physical changes: I was going to be fine.

I tried to push back any negative thoughts as I headed for the train, but I could feel the fear of what lay ahead rising from the back of my neck and pulsing into my temples. I decided to grab two Coronas for the train ride as I made my way to track 33. I thought it would be nice to drink a beer with Andrew, take the edge off as we watched the city speed by and away. I worked up a pretty good sweat rushing to the platform, with only a minute or so to spare. Clutching the beers in one hand, I speed-dialed Andrew. "Are you on the train?" I asked. "I'm about to hop on. Wanted to make sure you got on, too." The reception was bad underground, and Andrew was breaking up. "Should I get on this train or wait for the next one?" I asked.

I thought I heard him say he was getting on, so I raced into the first car and sat down. Immediately my phone rang, and it was Andrew asking, "Did you get on the train? Where are you?"

"I'm in the first car. Walk down through the . . ." Just as I was finishing my sentence, I felt the heat of an angry set of eyes glaring at me from behind a pair of glasses. ". . . train. I'm halfway down the aisle on the left."

As soon as I hung up, the man in glasses turned to face me, put his forefinger condescendingly to his lips, and said, "SSSHHHHHH!"

My temperature started to rise. There are few things that bother me more than being shushed as an adult, by an adult. I couldn't help it. "Sir, I was talking to my husband, trying to find him on the train. It's not as if I was in a deep conversation. That took all of fifteen seconds. My God."

But then my phone rang again.

As the man continued to glare at me, I repeated in a whisper, "I'm in the first car of the train. Come find me. I have to go now." Just then a prerecorded announcement filled the car. "A reminder to everyone on board: The first car on this train is the quiet car."

Okay, okay. The shushing man may have had his point. I'd broken the rules, but we hadn't even left the station yet, and I had been whispering for a few seconds. And then things took an unfortunate turn, because the man couldn't resist rubbing it in.

"See!" He snorted and pointed at me, saying loudly, "I told you so. If you want to talk, you need to leave this car." And that's when I completely, absolutely, 100 percent lost it. All of the emotion of the day, the loss of control I felt over my own body, the knowledge of the hell I was about to enter, and, ultimately, a tremendous fear of the unknown came crashing down on me. I can't recall ever doing anything like this before in my life, but I stood up and exploded.

"You, sir, are an asshole!" I shouted, adrenaline coursing through me. "Do you understand that I was trying to find my husband? Are you that miserable that you can't cut someone a fifteen-second break TO FIND HER HUSBAND? I hope you have a happy Thanksgiving, and don't forget, you are an ASSHOLE!" (I was tempted to add, *Oh, and by the way, I have cancer, and I just found out I'm facing eight rounds of chemotherapy*, but I resisted. I did, however, enunciate that second "ASSHOLE!" extra loudly as I grabbed my things—including my two beers—and tore out of the now not-so-quiet car. It occurred to me later that the other people in that car may have thought I was drunk or crazy, but I was way past caring.)

I walked down the aisles from car to car, my eyes tearing up, until I bumped into Andrew, who'd been racing the length of the train in the opposite direction.

"What happened?" he said. "What's wrong?"

Before I even finished my story, Andrew said, "Where is he? What does he look like?" He headed back the way I'd come.

Normally, I'm a lover, not a fighter. But a primal source of pride welled up inside me as I watched my husband go to defend my honor and tell off this smug middle-aged man. It was going to be awesome. *I don't care if we both get kicked off the train for it,* I thought. *In fact, I'll be proud of that, too!*

As I waited for Andrew to return, I imagined all the things he might be saying to the "shhh-er," and they were all satisfying.

When Andrew found his way back to me, he was smiling. "When I got to the first car, I asked loudly, 'Who's responsible for upsetting my wife?' And everyone pointed right at the man with the glasses." Then Andrew told me what he said to him, and I laughed out loud for the first time that afternoon. It was pretty much my speech verbatim, beginning with "Asshole" and ending with "Happy Thanksgiving." I had never heard anything sweeter.

We sat down and sipped our beers, and as I started to feel calmer, a train conductor walked over to us. *We're going to get booted,* I thought, and braced myself for one more jolt of tension. But then he smiled.

"I just wanted to tell you that if you hadn't said that to that man back there, I would've, on behalf of everyone in the car," he said. "I'm sorry he treated you like that, but some people are mean and angry. Please have a wonderful holiday."

And with that, I started to cry again. I'm fairly certain I cried more in these past four weeks than I had in my previous four decades.

As we settled into our seats and rode north, I realized that I was in for a long haul and that I needed to get a grip. Yes, I was terrified of all the misery to come and of leaving my daughters without a mother to guide them through life. I was afraid of losing control of my emotions and my dignity. And though I had faced down a fair amount of difficult stuff in my life, nothing had prepared me for this. But when I thought back to where I came from—my family and the way they'd always surrounded me with love and brought me up to work for what I wanted and to keep going no matter what—I realized that maybe I did, indeed, have the inner strength to make it through this year.

Chapter Four

A Sixth Sense

I am not a fearful person. In fact, as a reporter I fall more on the "willing to do just about anything" end of the spectrum. But I never thought of that as bravery. I did what was asked of me without thinking about it too much, mostly because I wanted to keep working but also because I've always craved new and exciting experiences.

I've gone ice road trucking in the Arctic Circle, where the ice is thick enough to handle the weight and speed of the vehicles for only three weeks a year. In 2011, after being "drown-proofed" by the U.S. Navy, I catapulted off an aircraft carrier in an F-18 and pulled 7 G's, breaking the sound barrier. For over a year, I reported out of a helicopter five days a week. I've crash-landed in a C-17 on a three-thousand-foot runway on a tiny Icelandic island in the middle of the North Atlantic, flown in Black Hawk and Huey helicopters, and even agreed to be a passenger in a single-engine Cessna piloted by a ten-year-old child. When I was twenty-five, a few years into my first job as a crime reporter, I witnessed an execution.

I never thought about the emotional or physical risks of these assignments. I was born with a fearless, independent spirit. My mom tells me that at the age of two, I'd stand at the front door of our apartment, banging on it and shouting, "I'ma go bye-bye." At age three, I'd purposefully get "lost" the moment we walked into any store. My mom would turn around to find me suddenly gone, and as soon as she started to race down the aisles looking for me, she would hear over the store speakers: "We have a lost little girl at the counter; could the parents of 'Amy' please come to the front of the store." My mom would rush up and find me there, usually with a lollipop from the cashier, smiling and having a great time with my new friend, not a care in the world. My mom says she sees that same little girl in me now, the one who can't wait to see what's around the corner, always looking for a new adventure. Before cancer, I never thought about dying. I've even joked that "my people," as in my family, live forever, which is only a *slight* exaggeration.

My dad is one of six and my mother is one of nine, German Catholics on both sides. My great-grandparents on my mother's side immigrated to Chicago in their teens, then moved to a cherry farm in Coloma, Michigan. My grandfather's first language was German. It's only a snapshot in my head, but one of my first memories is of sitting on my uncle Frank's lap, riding a tractor around the farm in Coloma. My grandpa on my father's side, Donald Robach, was the son of a housepainter and my grandma, Dorothy, was the daughter of a gas station owner. My dad's parents struggled financially, my grandpa working his way through his master's and Ph.D. in microbiology as an X-ray technician at the very hospital where I was born. My grandma stayed home to care for their rapidly growing family, four boys and two girls.

I was born in Lansing, in Sparrow Hospital, not far from the campus of Michigan State University. My parents were living in married-student housing when I came along. My dad is from St. Joseph, Michigan, a cute, Norman Rockwell kind of place on the shores of Lake Michigan. My mother lived across the river in Benton Harbor, a working-class town where even today the median income is less than half of what it is in St. Joe. Her father was a home builder, and my father's father became a microbiologist working for Whirlpool. My parents met in middle school at their church's youth group, and although the two families weren't very happy about how young my parents were on their wedding day, they eventually grew to love and respect their decision.

My grandmother on my mother's side—Willie Lee Parvin—grew up in Gulfport, Mississippi, and, oh, how she hates the name Willie! But when her mother was pregnant, her grandfather, William Stone, asked his daughter to name the baby after him. Unfortunately, the baby was a girl, so they named her Willie Lee. (For reasons I've never understood, they named her brother Shirley Austin. No doubt he was saying, "Don't call me Shirley!" long before the movie *Airplane!* came out. Smartly, he went by his initials—so we all knew him as Uncle S.A.)

My grandmother goes by "Lee," but when my grandfather wants to rile her up, he screams, "Willie Lee!" and she screams back, "Don't you call me that, Frank!"

Grandfather was in the Navy, stationed in Gulfport during World War II. He was actually engaged to another woman at the time, but then he met Lee at a USO event, and within three months they were married. He wrote a note to his fiancée, telling her he was sorry and, according to my mom, trying to get the ring back, an effort that predictably did not succeed. He convinced Lee to move to Michigan to be near his family, and once she settled in there, she made Southern goodies like grits, fried chicken, and mashed potatoes to go along with the braunschweiger, German sauerkraut, and potato salad. She doesn't have much of a Southern accent anymore, just a hint of a drawl.

Her father had been a farm-league baseball player, and when he didn't make it into the majors, he became a coal miner in Kentucky. After his appendix burst, he survived for several days in the hospital, until he told my grandmother, who was thirteen at the time, to go home and bake him a welcome-home cake. He was gone a few hours later. My great-grandmother moved the whole family back to Mississippi, where she became a seamstress and raised six children on her own. She died while my mom was pregnant with me, so I never knew her, but my mom said she was the toughest woman she'd ever met—a feminist before her time. So I guess you could say there's a family tradition of strong-willed women, with an equally strong work ethic.

My dad, much like his dad, juggled three jobs to earn his way through a bachelor's degree. My mom dropped out of community college, became a secretary at the MSU vet clinic, and devoted herself to raising two children; thanks to the Church's suggested rhythm method, my brother had come along when she was just twenty-one. She would eventually go back to get her degree and become a teacher.

We moved to Blacksburg, Virginia, shortly after Eric was born, so my dad could get his master's in microbiology at Virginia Tech. According to family lore, my own headstrong nature became evident not long after we arrived. At the age of three, I was at the sandbox outside married housing in Blacksburg, and I told my mom, "Tonight's Halloween."

"No," she said. "It's tomorrow."

I started whining, trying to convince her. "Mom, it's today, *they* said," I insisted, while pointing to the kids still playing outside.

"Amy, I think I know the calendar. It's not Halloween."

And yet, that night, as she was clearing the plates from dinner: *ding-dong.* "Trick or treat." The student-housing complex had decided to move the festivities up a day because today was Saturday.

"I told you," I said.

And, in a development that may come as no surprise to older siblings, after Eric was born, I tried to kill him. My mom said she once saw me pounce on my newborn brother in the same way I jumped all over my dad. But Eric and I became super-close. We made up a game called "mail": Players—just the two of us—wrote sweet letters and delivered them under each other's doors. Once, my brother asked me not to grow up and leave him, but what he wrote was "live" him. My mom still has it. (That was back in the day when he said he wanted to marry my mom.) Even though Eric's a high-powered doctor now, I see that same gentle nature in the way he treats his wife, Michelle, who was his college sweetheart, and their three boys.

When I was four, my dad got his first big job, working in St. Louis for Monsanto as what he dubbed a "lab rat." When we'd visit him in the office, he would do cool projects involving dry ice and mysterious liquids in glass beakers that turned different colors. I remember thinking my father was the smartest man in the world and proudly—and repeatedly—telling my kindergarten class, "My dad's a scientist."

Two years later, we bought a house in St. Peters, Missouri. If you looked up "suburb" in the dictionary, there would be a picture of 19 Craigwood Drive next to the entry. It looked like the *Brady Bunch* house, except it wasn't that big or that nice. It had three levels, all with low ceilings. The little living room and kitchen were decorated in shades of mustard and orange (it was the late seventies, after all). You could go downstairs to a small TV room or upstairs to the bedrooms, but you had to be careful not to barrel into anyone coming in the opposite direction, because the stairs were so narrow.

Our backyard abutted a forest. We spent many summers playing a game called "lost in the woods," where we'd pretend to be lost children, fending for ourselves, and our neighborhood friends would take on different characters. I was always Annie, naming my character after my favorite aunt, Ann. Eric always called himself Michael, perhaps after my dad. My character was older and wiser than my actual eight-year-old self, and Eric played a toddler, much younger than his six years. We spent hours and hours in our make-believe world. It was truly magical.

It was a game conceived out of necessity. During those long summer breaks, my mom worked at home for Monsanto, making graphics for presentations. Apparently we drove her crazy, constantly whining "Mom, we're bored, give us something to do." One day, she decided to lock us out. "Go play with each other and come back for lunch," she told us.

"But we're hot. We're thirsty," Eric and I pleaded.

"There's a hose. Figure it out," she said. And we did—and had the time of our lives.

Parents didn't worry so much about their kids back then, and nobody locked their doors. We rode our bikes all over the neighborhood. It seemed like nearly every house on our street had kids our age, and every summer we would all—and I mean everyone on our block—go on float trips in the Ozarks. We'd pitch tents, make big bonfires, and hike. Then we would hop in canoes, float down the river, and set up camp again. I realize now that this must've been a huge sacrifice for my mom, because she really appreciates a good hotel room, with a hot shower and clean toilet. She had to have been miserable. But that's the kind of love I grew up with.

The truth is, Mom gave up everything for my dad and us. She moved far away from her family and friends at the age of twenty-one. Most days, my dad drove our only car (a cinnamon-colored Chevette) to work, so she was stuck at home with two kids at her heels, unable to even go out and run errands. No doubt she worked through plenty of *How the hell did I get here?* demons.

And yet for us it was great. At least four times a year, we'd pile into our tiny car and drive six hours from St. Peters to Benton Harbor, Michigan, with my brother and me fighting the whole way! The cornfields of Illinois flying past my window, Stevie Nicks playing on the radio . . . those were the days. When we finally arrived at my grandparents' house, a modest four-bedroom ranch, there was never enough room for us all, but we packed in anyway and loved it. There were so many cousins (remember, my mom has eight siblings) that we would rush to "call" our space on the floor and mark our territory with our sleeping bags. My grandmother was always cooking, her way of showing love. Homemade mashed potatoes were her specialty. "There's no such thing as too much butter," she'd say.

My grandmother's house has always been full. Even today, she and Grandfather have a home in Atlanta with a basement apartment, and there's always some family member living down there. I don't believe they've ever had an empty nest, but my grandmother loves it. She lives for her children. That's her lifeblood.

When we were in St. Peters, my dad traveled a lot for work. He went to Europe and Asia, sometimes for weeks at a time. While he was away, my mom, my brother, and I spent a lot of time in our basement, a tiny, half-finished room with thin wood paneling and a big couch. The main attraction was the TV, complete with an Atari set, but we also headed down there every time our town's tornado siren sounded—and that happened a lot. I joke that I've spent at least five years of my life in tornado position, rolled into a ball with my hands clasped around the back of my neck. We had drills all the time in school and a couple of close calls at home. Our house was up on a small ridge, and I remember stepping out of that basement once after hearing a twister in the distance, to find the homes below us destroyed. I'll never forget the greenish-yellow color the sky turns right before a tornado strikes. The sirens go off, and you hit the basement. That's the way it is when you live in the tornado belt.

My mom was very strict, and we could only watch certain TV shows at certain times. She'd allow *The Love Boat* and *The Dukes of Hazzard*, and occasionally we'd sneak in *Dallas* on Friday nights. What Eric and I really loved, though, were scary movies. My mom never allowed them—an easy rule to enforce, at least in theory, because we didn't have cable or own a VCR when I was in grade school. But that didn't stop me. On those long summer days, I would head down to my best friend's house, which had HBO, and watch all the scary movies I wanted. I was in third grade when my friend Carrie Gibson and I watched *Poltergeist,* and I was never the same. Yes, I hated how afraid I was of my closet every night, sweating out liquid fear in my bed, but I also loved the adrenaline rush I felt while watching ghosts and ax murderers hunt their victims. I was addicted. I remember going to my next-door neighbor Lori Mims's house to watch Jason and his ski mask in *Friday the 13th*. It would be pretty hard to find a scary movie

I haven't seen. The original *Psycho* with Tony Perkins. *The Omen* with Gregory Peck. *The Exorcist*. *The Shining*. It must be something about my metabolism. I describe myself as an adrenaline junkie (which also explains what I do for a living). But I also think scary movies have always helped me escape from my real life. Even when things aren't going well, they could be worse—as in, *a demon could be possessing me!*

By the time I got to high school, I'd stay up late on weekends to watch *The Twilight Zone* and *Alfred Hitchcock Presents*. And when my girlfriends slept over—nearly every Saturday night—we would go to Blockbuster to rent as many scary movies as we could carry. The first movie Andrew and I ever saw together was *The Haunting in Connecticut*. He didn't tell me until later that he hates scary movies. (Thankfully, he liked *me*!)

When I got to be ten or eleven, I started reading horror books. My favorite author was Stephen King. Mom would take us to the library— who could resist the cool air-conditioning, a relief from the unbearably steamy St. Louis summer days?—and I'd walk straight to "K." She would say, "Really? You could read anything, and that's what you want to read?"

"Yep." I read all those books, and twenty years later I had the thrill of a lifetime when I got to interview King for NBC. I told him, "You ruined my childhood with Pennywise the clown [from *It*]."

His response: "Good!" He had a big grin on his face.

My daughters have the same addiction—they can't stop reading and watching the scary stuff. Andrew pulls his hair out, because he and his boys hate it, so we wait until they're downstairs watching soccer. (Andrew briefly played for the L.A. Galaxy, so it's an understandable obsession for my guys; since being married to Andrew, I've learned that there is a soccer game on some channel at any given hour of the day.) Then we pile into my bed and click over to whatever scary movie we have on deck.

———

MY BROTHER AND I went to a small rural Catholic elementary school with only forty students per grade. I was very independent, but Eric was a classic second child, so he liked that his big sister was around to look after him at school.

At St. Elizabeth Ann Seton, anytime you got sick you had to go see Sister Greisedich to get permission to go home. One day I developed a fever, and Sister called my mom to come pick me up. She then sent word over to Eric's teacher to tell him not to look for me but to wait for his normal pickup in the parking lot when the bell rang. Mom and I were home for all of thirty minutes when Sister called, saying that Eric was now "sick." This happened more than once, and each time, my mom would go back and retrieve him. It must have been enormously frustrating to her at the time, but now we both gently tease him about it.

Eric and I were both straight-A students, but I could never stop chatting, and my conduct grades weren't up to my academic marks. I was the one passing notes and whispering during class. But all the sisters had to do was look at me in their stern, quiet way, and I would die a thousand deaths. I hated for anyone to be upset with me. One day in sixth grade, I couldn't stop laughing, and then I couldn't stop hiccupping, because when I laugh, I get the hiccups. It's a Robach trait that I've unfortunately passed on to my daughters. Sister Patricia said to me, "Miss Robach, come here."

I was mortified already, but I walked up to her desk and stood there for a moment. She raised her hands, looked me in the eye, and slammed them down hard on the desk. As the heat rose in my cheeks, she continued to stare at me for what must have been fifteen seconds; the silence was killing me, because I did not know what she was going to do or say next. She finally smiled and said, "Good. Looks like I cured you. Go back to your seat."

The nuns at our very traditional school were, for the most part, kind and giving. Some of the priests were far more intimidating. I remember feeling so frightened when Father Marshall (who would make you stand for the entire class if he caught you yawning) taught us about purgatory and limbo. I was terrified by the idea that if a baby died before being baptized, he or she couldn't go to heaven. How could the God I was learning about banish a newborn baby to a place called limbo? I certainly learned the meaning of "God-fearing," but I didn't like the implication that the primary reason to do good things was out of fear of repercussions in the afterlife. Much later, when I was working as a reporter in the Deep South, I started questioning more of what I'd been taught. I always hated it when people who had survived some mass tragedy would say, "The Lord saved me." As if "the Lord" chose them to survive and let others die. I always thought that was awfully narcissistic. I didn't see how God would play favorites.

I consider myself a spiritual person, and I believe in the afterlife and I believe in God, but I can't say that I'm a big fan of organized religion. I give to Catholic Charities, and I send my kids to Catholic school because I think there's immense value in reinforcing their moral foundation outside the home. I also love that my kids are learning about the histories and traditions of all religions and that their school takes a softer approach to some of the teachings I struggled to understand as a child. For instance, I'm certain my daughters only know "limbo" as a fun party game. And I would never undo my Catholic upbringing and education, because it strengthened my moral compass and contributed to who I am today. As for the guilt and humility associated with the Church—well, I believe those can be developmentally important. You *should* feel ashamed sometimes, if you've done something wrong.

Of course, Catholic school didn't teach us about sex, but truth be told I was never all that curious. I'd seen men and women kissing, mostly my parents, and my reaction was pretty much, *So what?* It never occurred to me that kissing led to anything else.

My brother, however, was always insanely curious about anything having to do with biology. While I was over in the horror stacks at the library—and every now and then back to *Little House on the Prairie* or *Anne of Green Gables*—he had his nose in medical journals. After my friend Stacey Schneider died, he found out that sores that don't heal and bruises that won't go away are among the first symptoms of leukemia, and he convinced himself he had it.

When I was in fourth grade and Eric was in second, we were on one of those interminable trips from St. Peters to Michigan, a long day in the Chevette, and we were somewhere south of Chicago when my brother asked about how babies were made.

My parents glanced at each other. Mom tried to hedge: "Oh, you know . . . two cells get together and they form a baby." But my brother the science geek wasn't going to be dismissed that easily.

"But how do the two cells get together? I don't understand. How does the dad cell get with the mom cell?"

That was the point at which my dad started laughing and pulled into a gas station to fill up the tank.

My mom looked at him through the car window and said, "Really? You're going to do this to me?"

I could feel the awkwardness filling up that tiny car, and I remember thinking that maybe I didn't want to know how the two cells got together. But Eric kept pushing, and eventually my mom said, "Fine. You know what? I'm going to tell you."

And she did, in PG-13 detail.

My brother listened, nodded his head serenely, and said, "Now it makes sense."

I was mortified. I put my hands over my mouth and closed my eyes, shaking my head. "No, that just can't be true," I said, feeling blindsided. I was so upset that my mother later said she wished she'd punted the conversation for a couple of years. For months after "the talk," I looked at every couple and counted how many kids they had. I knew that sex was only for procreation, so the number of children you had equaled the number of times you'd had sex. That meant my mom and dad had done it twice. One day I looked at my grandmother and thought, *Nine times!* Whenever I saw somebody with kids, I couldn't help myself: My mind instantly did the sex math.

There were boys in my school, but they sat at separate lunch tables, and the sisters kept us apart throughout the rest of the day. The effort was wasted on my behalf, because I thought boys were simply gross. I was on the nerdy side through middle school. It didn't help that I still looked nine at thirteen: no chest, no hips, zero curves. I was a competitive gymnast from second grade until I switched to cheerleading at fourteen. So for six years I spent much of my free time at a gym, and toward the end I was putting in twenty hours a week.

After my first year of gymnastics, I joined an elite team, and we traveled around the state to compete. The coach suggested I take private lessons with him to sharpen my skills, but my parents could barely afford the monthly class bill, so I stuck with team practice four or five days a week.

The gymnastics coach became more than just a coach; he was like a second father to me. He told me that he loved me. He would say, "Amy, wear your hair in French braids for me. You look beautiful when your hair is back," and I'd beg my mom to braid it before practice. At the end of class, he would go down the line of girls for a hug and a quick kiss on the lips. He was a churchgoing family man with a wife and family, so everyone thought it was fatherly affection, if a little intense. The only time my mom expressed any hesitation was when the coach had team sleepovers at his house. She only allowed me to attend parent-chaperoned sleepovers at the gym, not the ones in his home, and I would tell her that I was being left out, that my other teammates all went. But it turned out that she was right to be skeptical.

Life was busy but settled into a comfortable, ordinary rhythm— school, gymnastics, homework, church—until one day in sixth grade. I was on the beam and the coach was spotting me for a front flip when he got this strange, fixated look that made me feel extremely uncomfortable. He was half smiling, and his eyes seemed to look through me. It was creepy, as if he were possessed. I felt a wave of fear and blurted out, "Stop looking at me like that."

But he kept staring as if in a trance, and I started to shout, "If you don't stop looking at me like that, I'm getting off this beam right now." He didn't, though, and tears welled up in my eyes. He looked menacing—nothing like the fatherly figure I had worked so hard to impress all these years. I jumped down and ran to the front office to call my mother. I was crying by now and tried to explain what had happened, but it was hard to make her understand what was so *off* about that moment. She said, "You're probably just overreacting, honey. He is your coach, and you shouldn't speak to him that way. But Dad is on his way to pick you up, so you don't have to go back there now." I waited in the lobby, feeling very confused and a little scared.

Two weeks later, my parents came to school and took me out of class. They walked me out to the car, and I knew something very serious had happened. I thought someone had died. "Your gymnastics coach has been arrested," my mom said. "And we need to ask you a serious question."

They had looks of concern on their faces like I'd never seen before. I braced myself for what was next.

"Did he ever touch you?"

"No."

They still looked so worried that I started to cry. "I don't understand. What's going on?"

"He's been charged with hurting one of your teammates," they said.

A girl had come forward and said he'd molested her. It was all over the news, and after a few days, several other girls came forward with similar stories. According to them, it happened during those sleepovers and private lessons.

I thought I was going to throw up. I remembered all of those hugs and kisses and the French braids. I felt ashamed that I had felt any affection toward a man who was accused of this. I can still see his mug shot in the *St. Louis Post-Dispatch,* and it makes me physically ill to this day. We were all shaken but also grateful that my mom had trusted her gut and not allowed me to attend any of the sleepovers. Still, she felt terrible about how she had responded to my phone call. "When you feel something strange or weird, when your body tells you something is wrong, trust yourself," she said. "And I promise to always listen to you, too." It's something I say to my own daughters all the time.

The gym shut down, and for a while it seemed my whole world had disappeared with it. I was depressed and felt betrayed. I couldn't think about what might have happened to my friends, my teammates, the ones who were too scared to come forward. It was too terrible.

Unfortunately, it was only the beginning of a rough year. Just before Christmas, my dad told us he was going to quit his job and go into the home-building business with my mom's father and brothers. We were going to have to leave St. Peters, my friends, and everything I'd known since I was four years old. "To go where?" I asked.

"Snellville, Georgia."

"Snellville! You've got to be kidding me." My grandparents had moved to the town, right outside Atlanta, a couple of years before, and now my parents were investing their life savings and what would have been our college money in this new venture. My dad knew nothing about construction, but he was fed up with having to travel so much for Monsanto. So we packed everything into a U-Haul and moved in with my grandparents.

I was twelve (but still looked like a third-grader), and I was being transplanted from a small Catholic school in the Midwest to a huge public middle school down South. I went from wearing a uniform every day, with no makeup or nail polish, to a place where the girls all had Jordache jeans, winged hair, and blue eyeliner. They all spoke with a Southern drawl and said "y'all" and "fixin' to go." I tried to fit in, but I couldn't shake "sneakers" and "you guys." It was a culture shock of epic proportions.

I vividly remember my first day at Five Forks Middle School. I'd never had to think about clothes before, and my mom and I thought it would be adorable if I wore a red-and-white pinstriped shirt, complete with a Peter Pan collar and bow. I had this little bob and glasses, and the next year I added braces to the mix, along with a bad perm. It was the first of many classic "sitting alone in the cafeteria" moments, being snubbed by the mean girls. I desperately wanted them to like me. I was, and still am, a people person, and there's nothing I hate more than being alone.

One boy in particular, Greg, tormented me relentlessly. He called me "Skeeter," because he said I had mosquito bites for boobs, and he repeated it constantly, as loud as he could. I was utterly mortified and humiliated. That first year in Georgia was so bad, I cried myself to sleep every night, literally, and I'm sure I was clinically depressed. I eventually even got mono. My mom felt so bad she let me get my ears pierced, but my dad was tough. He'd say, "Buck up and go to school!" In retrospect I realize he had to be incredibly stressed, too, living with his in-laws after quitting a profession he loved and risking his life savings. I wasn't helping things by frequently vocalizing my misery.

It was six months before we found our own place, just down the road from my grandparents, and all that time I slept on the floor of my aunt Ann's bedroom. I know I annoyed her immensely—I was a sixth-grader and she was a senior in high school—but I worshipped her. One day I was staring at her and said, "Ann, you're prettier than Marcia Brady." It was the highest compliment I could offer at the time. We still use that line today when we want a good laugh.

Despite my trouble at school, it felt good to be close to my aunts and uncles. Even though they're my mom's siblings, they're closer in age to Eric and me. Uncle Stephen was so good with us. Just seven years my senior, he would come up with interesting art projects, bake cookies, and play board games. My family's love got me through, and within a year everything was better. I was accepted into the Atlanta School of Gymnastics, a very renowned club, and I started back into a demanding practice regimen, which gave me structure and purpose. ASG was hard core—I remember watching elite gymnast Kristie Phillips, who was touted as the "New Mary Lou" (as in Retton) by *Sports Illustrated,* train there while she was traveling through the Atlanta area. But a year into the program, when my mom asked, "Is she good enough to make the Olympics?" my coach flatly said, "No." The truth hurt, but it was also a relief. It came at a time when I was making friends, and spending thirty hours a week at the gym wasn't great for my social life. When I quit a few weeks later, I felt free. That's when I tried out for cheerleading, and because I was a good gymnast, I made the team.

It had taken me a full year of struggling to make friends and fit in, but this grim period helped me develop the skills I'd use later in life. Unbeknownst to me, I was learning how to walk into a newsroom, accept that people might be difficult initially, and then win them over and make friends. I was learning to keep a positive attitude even when I was scared, alone, and feeling slightly bullied. I cheered for the next two years, until I found my true passion: musical theater.

Meanwhile, the construction business was not going as well as planned. The company wasn't making any money, and my parents were worried and stressed. They were struggling with finances and dealing with all the relationship issues that arise when you go into business with family. Then we experienced another trauma that put business problems—*any* problems, for that matter—into perspective.

It happened on the Fourth of July, the summer between eighth and ninth grade, when I was just fourteen. At this point, nearly our entire extended family had moved to Atlanta to be close to my grandparents. Even my grandmother's sister, Aunt Joyce, and her husband, Jack, had come down from Missouri, settling in on a beautiful farm in Monroe, Georgia, not far from us. To welcome them and their daughter, also named Amy, we decided to have a big picnic for the entire family at Briscoe Park in Snellville. There must have been thirty of us, because we took up an entire section of the park.

It was always fun hanging out with my aunts and uncles and cousins, but that year all I really cared about was whether or not my neighbor would be at the park to watch the fireworks. His name was Mike Oleksinski. He was two years older than me, tall and thin with brown hair and an adorable smile. I had a *huge* crush on him, so I spent hours getting ready, just in case. We didn't have much money, and I usually wore Aunt Ann's hand-me-downs or something we found on the final-markdown sale rack. But we'd been at the mall a few weeks earlier and my mom said, "Let's buy a new outfit for the Fourth." I almost never got new clothes, so I was thrilled, and we'd picked out some for my mom, too—something she rarely indulged in, either.

That morning I woke up excited to wear my new outfit, so I was completely caught off guard when I opened my drawer and felt a strange sensation. My stomach dropped and I thought, *You will never want to put these clothes on again after today*. I immediately felt embarrassed. I didn't believe in premonitions, and no one in my family did, either, so I tried to pretend it didn't happen. But a feeling of unease lingered in the back of my head, and I had to consciously push it out of my thoughts several times that day. As much as I tried to convince myself it was nonsense, I knew there was something to it. Since that day, I've experienced many similar moments—I just know when something particularly good or bad is coming around the bend. Call it intuition or a sixth sense, but I now trust that feeling when it happens.

By midafternoon we were at the park, Mom and I were dressed in our new Casual Corner outfits, and any dark thoughts had vanished. After we devoured an epic picnic, my cousins, my brother, and I took off to walk around the lake and look for our friends. About ten minutes into our scouting, the skies started to darken, and when the first few raindrops fell, we ran for cover under a nearby pavilion. I did *not* want to get my new outfit wet, and, perhaps more important, I didn't want to get my hair wet (I was still hoping to run into Mike Oleksinski).

Within a few minutes, at least twenty people had pushed in together with us under the pavilion. We were watching the clouds quickly turn from a dull gray to an ominous midnight black when a massive bolt of lightning streaked out of the sky and struck the ground only a few feet in front of us. There was a deafening boom and crackle, and everyone screamed. I felt electricity tingling in the air, and then the rain came down in a biblical deluge.

After the shock of the lightning bolt faded, we began to laugh nervously and joke about what a close call it had been. Minutes later, though, we began to see ambulances and fire trucks pulling into the park, emergency lights flashing. Just beneath the pounding noise of the rain, which was also blurring the view, we could hear sirens and people yelling nearby. My brother, who's always been the worrier in the family, turned to me and said, "That looks really close to where we were. Where those flashing lights are—that's right where we were sitting."

I said, "Oh, come on, you actually think our family got struck by lightning?"

"I don't know, but I'm going to check."

He ran off in the rain, and I stayed behind with my cousin Laura. "I'm not getting my hair wet," I told her.

We stayed there another five minutes, but as each second ticked by and my brother didn't return, I got the feeling that something was terribly wrong. I eventually pushed myself into the pounding rain, my heart beating through my chest. I was getting soaked to the bone and I didn't care. As I approached the scene, everything slowed, and I saw my uncle Ken stumbling around, saying, "Where am I?" Then I saw another man slumped near a tree. I didn't recognize him, because he was so bloated and blue. EMTs were trying to restart his heart with a defibrillator.

That's when I heard my mom scream, "I can't feel my legs!" She was on the ground, surrounded by EMTs and my aunt Patty. To my right, I saw my dad on the ground with a group of EMTs working on him, as well, my uncle Paul by his side. I had only been on the scene for about thirty seconds when I fell to my knees in the middle of all the chaos, my mouth hanging open in disbelief. I put both of my hands to my head to try to steady myself; I felt dizzy. I saw my brother in the distance, crying, and that's when Aunt Patty came running up to me and said, "Amy, both of your parents have been struck by lightning. We need to get you out of here. I don't want you to see this."

Everything was a blur. I don't even know who led me out of the park and into the parking lot, but all of a sudden I was whisked into a stranger's van. My family was so focused on trying to help at the scene that they asked another family to take us out of the rain and out of sight. I know they were all doing the best they could in the midst of the shock and trauma, but it was horrible not to know what was happening with my parents. I kept trying to climb out of the van, and Uncle Paul kept saying, "Get back in the van, Amy, get back in the van." The family who owned the van was praying with us, and Eric and I were bawling. "I just want to know what's going on," I said. But we were completely shut out. I kept thinking the worst, imagining myself orphaned at fourteen. *Who will raise me? My grandparents? One of my aunts or uncles?* I was crying so hard, my chest hurt.

It seemed like hours before my grandmother and grandfather finally came over and said, "Your mom and dad are both alive; they're doing okay, and they are headed to the hospital. We'll take you there now."

I found out later that the unrecognizable man I saw first was my uncle Jack. He'd been leaning against the tree when it took a direct hit. My parents had been holding lawn chairs over their heads and calling for all the kids to come, while everyone was running around and packing up. Uncle Jack took the brunt of the bolt, but my parents were thrown nearly twenty feet across the ground. Their tennis shoes were blown off their feet, and their clothes were singed to their bodies. My dad initially lost consciousness, and my mom couldn't move from the waist down.

We waited in the hospital lobby for hours, and finally, sometime after midnight, my grandparents convinced the doctors to let Eric and me quickly see our parents. The doctors said my parents were extremely lucky but would stay in the ICU overnight. I didn't get back to my grandparents' house until well after 1:00 A.M., and when I started to undress, I suddenly remembered that awful feeling I'd had eighteen hours earlier, putting on my new outfit. I thought about the medics cutting off my mom's clothes, which had been burned to her body. I remember thinking, *Oh no, Mom's brand-new outfit.* I'm sure it was a coping mechanism: If I worried about the money my mom had spent on that outfit, I wouldn't have to think about her dying.

But that night, trying to go to sleep at my grandparents' house was nearly impossible. I was so afraid something would happen to my parents overnight in the hospital and I would never see them again. As for my premonition, I kept that to myself for years and years, eventually telling my parents about it after I went to college. I was pleasantly surprised when they told me they believed me. Somehow I thought they would think I was making it up, and there were times *I* even thought I was making it up, but I know in my heart I wasn't. Acknowledging and accepting my intuition has been a struggle for me, but I am getting better as experience teaches me to trust it time and again. I never wore those clothes after that day. I hid them at the bottom of my drawer, until they eventually made their way to the pile we collected once a year for Goodwill.

My mom was in the hospital for several days, my dad spent one night, and my uncle Jack didn't make it. The medics revived him on the scene, but he had spent too much time deprived of oxygen, and his brain slowly swelled. He died a week after the accident. It was incredibly sad—he was only in his mid-sixties, a great husband and father, and a very gentle and kind man.

My dad had stitches on the top of his head, where the bolt struck him. His heartbeat was irregular, and every muscle in his body ached. My mom slowly regained feeling and full mobility, although years later she had to have back surgery. She had internal bleeding and muscle aches, but the bolt left something so remarkable behind that the nurses kept coming in to look at her: My mom was marked with a second-degree burn—like a tattoo—of a lightning bolt (a jagged line, just like you see in the sky). You could see where it had entered under her right arm—she was holding that lawn chair over her head—and streaked across her torso. There was even an exit wound on her left thigh. It took years for it to go away, and every time she got hot, the lightning bolt came back, angry and red. Both my parents had a really tough time walking afterward, and for the rest of the summer they slept on our downstairs couch, because it was too painful to navigate the stairs to their bedroom. It took them an entire year to fully recover.

The incident got massive local news coverage. A family getting struck by lightning—now, that's a lead story! I remember thinking it was so cool that all the reporters wanted to talk to us, but my mom was incredibly embarrassed. She kept saying, "What kind of idiot stands out in the middle of a thunderstorm and gets struck by lightning?"

She hated the attention, so someone suggested that the best way to make it go away was to pick one outlet and do an extensive interview. My parents decided on *The Atlanta Journal-Constitution*. A reporter and a photographer came into my mom's hospital room, where all four of us were waiting nervously. The photographer took pictures, and then the interview began. My mom was adamant that none of us tell him about the lightning bolt seared onto her body.

"I'm a freak show," she'd say. "I belong in the circus."

At some point, the reporter asked, "What did you think happened when the lightning bolt struck?"

Mom replied honestly. "I thought a bomb went off. I thought it was the end of the world. I don't know. I just knew that all of a sudden I was on the ground and I couldn't feel anything."

The next morning, the headline read, WOMAN THINKS IT'S END OF THE WORLD. My mom was mortified. Her daughter, the future reporter, however, cut out all the newspaper articles and saved them.

That next year, in ninth grade, I wrote a piece about the ordeal and entered it in the Gwinnett County Mosaic Writing Fair. I won—one of the few times I'd ever gotten first place at anything. Even in all my years as a competitive gymnast, I always seemed to come in second or third. I was thrilled but also knew that the subject matter couldn't be beat.

THE EXPERIENCE CHANGED our family forever, as tragedies do. I never fully acknowledged how afraid I had been, the trauma of those heart-stopping hours in a stranger's van when I wasn't sure if my parents were going to survive. I was just fourteen and was not comfortable talking about those fears, and I didn't want to admit how vulnerable I felt, so I buried it. My mom also struggled to move forward with ease. Her new default outlook was: *No one is safe, and lightning can strike twice.* I can still see her running out to stop my brother's baseball game mid-inning because she'd heard thunder. We suddenly understood that anything can happen in a split second to anyone, anytime, anywhere.

Not many people get struck by lightning and live to tell their stories. My uncle paid the ultimate price, but my parents got a second chance. I'd like to say we made a point after that tragedy to appreciate each and every day on this earth, but that is no easy task. For me, it wasn't until I heard a doctor tell me I had breast cancer that I decided to live differently, to live with gratitude.

Chapter Five

All Grown Up by Age Twenty-Three

I spent my high school years at Brookwood High School in Snellville, Georgia, alongside twenty-four hundred other students—that's about six hundred kids per grade. It was easy to get lost in the shuffle. I tried to span several different cliques and have a variety of friends. I was a good student, I took AP classes and was a member of the Beta Club and the National Honor Society, and I eventually switched from cheerleading to the performing arts. Theater became my obsession. I auditioned for every school play but didn't start landing roles until my junior and senior years. Aunt Patty and Uncle Ken were the theater directors for the high school, and they did their best not to show any favoritism. In fact, they went out of their way. I tried not to take it personally when I didn't land Ado Annie in *Oklahoma!* my senior year. I did manage to play Elizabeth in Mary Shelley's *Frankenstein* later that semester. It was probably more up my alley anyway, given my fascination with the abomination, but there's nothing quite like your mom's sister directing you on how to kiss your fellow lead in a love scene.

By now I definitely liked boys, but I never really had a serious boyfriend. My girlfriends were on the Homecoming Court each year. They dated hunky football and basketball stars, and I was the friend who got invited to fill in as necessary on double dates.

I didn't even get asked to my senior prom—I had to ask a friend who went to neighboring Tucker High School. I was very self-conscious about my looks. I was still underdeveloped and awkward around boys. My parents always told me I was beautiful, but they were *my parents,* so they had to think that, right? They also made a point not to focus on my looks, because they wanted to raise a sweet, smart young woman who was appreciated for her brains instead. I knew I had a good head on my shoulders, though, and that's where I found my strength. I also knew I was a kind person and a hard worker.

I started a neighborhood babysitting business when I was thirteen, and the week I turned sixteen I set out to find my first real job. I worked part-time at a local party-supply store during the school year, and by summer I began to work at Rich's department store. I worked there every summer and every Christmas and also part-time during school. My mom agreed to let me work twenty hours a week, only if my grades didn't slip.

I made sure to stay on top of it all, because nothing made me happier than having a job. I loved being independent, working hard, and getting a paycheck. It was also my excuse to drive the family car: a 1987 silver Chevrolet Celebrity, which I affectionately called "the Leb."

Money was tight, and I remember hearing my parents fight about it. The construction business was still not working out, and eventually my dad went back to doing what he did (and loved) best—being a microbiologist—even though it meant a lot of traveling again. He found a job at Wayne Farms, a division of Continental Grain, as the vice president for food safety. He'd taken the big gamble to try to improve our lot, and luckily we all came out okay in the end, but I was at an impressionable age. I must have internalized the fear of not knowing whether or not we'd be able to pay the bills, so I never asked for extras, like money to go on the class trip to D.C. Not having everything handed to me shaped me tremendously, and with time I became grateful for the lesson in self-sufficiency. I continued to work at Rich's in the summers through college. I switched departments all the time: From handbags to accessories to menswear, I sold it all.

By this time, my aunt Ann had gone off to the University of Georgia to get her degree in broadcast journalism. Eventually she would become a main anchor at the NBC station in the Tri-Cities area of Tennessee and inspire me to follow in her footsteps.

Our career paths were blazed by my grandmother. She'd nudged Ann to be a journalist, because that's what she'd always dreamed of becoming herself but had been able to attend only one semester at Perkinston College in Gulfport, Mississippi. My grandmother had saved her money from working at her uncle's ice cream parlor during the summers and also worked part-time in the college president's office, doing secretarial work. Still, she ran out of money after her first semester and had to return home. She was extremely disappointed but had no other choice. There was no federal student-loan program back in the 1940s.

My grandmother pushed me to enter speech contests and to audition for plays, musicals, and commercials in the Atlanta area. She'd clip tryout announcements from the paper and send them to me. "Amy, you should go for this; you'd be perfect," she'd write.

All the women in my family were very strong and loving, and incredible role models. My mother gave up her dreams to take care of her children the same way my grandmother had, and she wanted me to experience more: a career, freedom, independence. She always discouraged boyfriends, and her mantra was, "You don't need to have kids until you're much older." (Remember, she had me at nineteen.) Even though she went back to school to become a teacher, it wasn't her dream career, and she found a creative outlet in community theater. She was talented. I remember seeing her in *Fiddler on the Roof* and *Anything Goes* and listening to her practice her solos day and night. But she poured her real energy and creativity into helping me develop any talent I might have. I loved my parents very much, and I wanted to please them, to make them proud. Their expectations were high. Of course I felt pressure, but I relished the challenge.

My parents were the strictest of any of my friends'. My curfew was eleven o'clock until I was a senior, and I had to pick one night, either Friday or Saturday, to go out. I couldn't go out both nights, because, as Mom liked to say, "I don't want to worry about you more than I have to." It was a very German Catholic mentality: Less is more, and don't speak unless spoken to. But at the same time I was encouraged to play the French horn, to be a gymnast, to take voice and acting lessons. My mom drove me all around town to make sure I had every opportunity to be anything I wanted to be. She also wanted me to have financial independence, something she and my grandmother, who'd given birth to ten children by the time she turned forty, never had. (Aunt Ann was a surviving twin—her identical sister, Laura, died within hours of birth.)

Good grades were a given. I don't think my brother made a single B the entire time he was in school, from kindergarten to college. I believe I had three or four. Still, neither of us applied to any of the more selective schools like Harvard or Yale, or even Duke or Vanderbilt. We didn't think in those terms, partly because of the cost—my folks didn't want us to be saddled with student loans—but also because they didn't want us far from home. Happily, we both got academic scholarships to the University of Georgia, and my mom had a hard enough time when I moved to Athens, forty-five minutes away!

Now I complain: "Mom, do you know what it's like? My husband went to Dartmouth, his brother and sister both went to Harvard, his dad went to Harvard, his mom went to Wellesley, my brother-in-law went to Brown—and I went to number five on the list of top-ten party schools!" But the fact is, I loved Georgia, and it was the perfect school for me. In addition to the half scholarship I had from the university based on my SAT scores and grades, I had a journalism scholarship I'd applied for and won and another scholarship from a private company based on an essay contest on journalism.

My parents wanted us to earn everything we got, and I thank them for that. During my first year in college, I had to take the bus to class and ask friends for rides back home. I didn't get a car until my junior year.

While at UGA, both my brother and I worked for an older gentleman named John Wilkins, a businessman who lived near campus and sold paper products out of his home. While the cheap college-kid labor was great, he mostly enjoyed having young people around him in his old age, I believe. There were four or five of us there at any given time, and he always found something for us to do. My dad came to Athens to meet him first, face-to-face, and then gave us the green light. We ran errands for John, wrote thank-you notes for him, and bought everything he needed, from gifts to groceries. Eric helped him with his computer. We made five dollars an hour. At the end of the day, we'd write ourselves a check and he'd sign it. Years later, when one of the news magazines ran a centerfold ad for MSNBC with me front and center, he cut it out, framed it, and mailed it to me. I still have it in my office.

During my freshman year in Athens, I shared a tiny dorm room in Boggs Hall with my best friend from high school, Ashley Curl. By the time I was a junior, I had moved into a six-hundred-square-foot, three-bedroom, one-bathroom apartment with five girls. My parents gave me two hundred dollars a month for rent and forty dollars a week for groceries. "I'm not paying for your entertainment-slash-beer money," my mother would say. If I wanted to go out to dinner or a concert or buy new clothes, I was on my own.

Just because I was living with girls didn't mean things were tidy. I am a neat freak, and living with roommates meant crawling over old pizza boxes and having to put up with cockroaches and dirty dishes in the sink. I was juggling journalism classes, a poli-sci minor, and an internship at WNGM TV-34 in Athens on a program called *Mornings with Meg.* Yes, mornings—which meant I had to get up at 3:00 A.M., about the time my roommates came stumbling in for the night. I did my fair share of partying my first two years of school, but now I was irritated, and I'm sure I annoyed them by being holier than thou, so eventually I called the tidiest person I know other than my mom: my brother. Senior year I moved in with Eric. Two of his fraternity brothers lived with us, and together we had the cleanest, quietest apartment on the block.

I never rushed a sorority, because I didn't like the concept of people asking me what my dad did for a living and judging me for how I looked and what I wore. I know the Greek system is a great way to find your place in a big university, and it is huge at UGA, but it wasn't the right fit for me. Plus, sorority dues are expensive, and I would have had to foot the bill. I just didn't have the money.

I love the South, and when I go back home I crank up country music on the car stereo and go to Georgia Bulldog football games, but some part of me always felt like a fish out of water. My academic passion was English. I loved literature and writing. I still adored theater, too. But none of those seemed like pursuits with steady job prospects, so I got a degree in broadcast journalism. The University of Georgia's Henry W. Grady College of Journalism is a first-rate program ("home of the Peabody Awards"), and it didn't take long before I knew I was exactly where I was supposed to be.

The best thing about the program was the broadcast-news course senior year. They limited enrollment to around forty people; every day we put on a live newscast, which was beamed into every dorm room at five in the afternoon. So while I was still taking classes for my degree, I was out in the community covering stories—and that's when I truly caught the journalism bug.

My first big story was about the death of a student, who happened to be a beautiful model. She'd been living in an apartment off campus, and she overdosed on Ecstasy. This was before cellphones and the Internet made tracking people down much easier, so I found her address in the phone book and drove out there.

It was about twenty-four hours after she'd died, and when I pulled up I saw a man carrying out furniture and putting it into the back of a pickup. I took a deep breath and walked up to him and said, "Sir. I'm so sorry to be here. My name is Amy Robach, and I'm with University News. Are you related to this young woman?"

He said, "I'm her father."

My heart was pounding, and I said, "I'm so sorry to ask you this, but I want to do a story about what happened. If we do a piece, it will go into every dorm room at the University of Georgia tonight, and if it stops one person from doing drugs, maybe her death can serve a purpose."

He looked at me with tears in his eyes and said, "Okay. I'll do it."

So we sat down, and within minutes we were both crying. It struck me what an unbelievable responsibility and honor it is to be able to tell people's stories and, if you do your job well, to know you can change someone else's life with that story. Just one person. If one person said no to drugs after that day, that was enough.

It was then that I knew to my core that I wanted to be a journalist. I loved theater, but here the drama was real life, and there was nothing as incredible as capturing those unscripted moments. I love feeling an intense bond with someone I've just met, someone who has entrusted his or her story to me. I love being a force for change and feeling the power of communication, too, but mostly I love the connection.

About this time, I started to connect with boys, or at least realize they sort of liked me. Up until college, I was the insecure girl who didn't feel like a woman yet. After all those years of being underdeveloped, it was hard to shake that "Skeeter" feeling from middle school.

But I *had* changed. I had grown into my body and no longer resembled a nine-year-old boy. I was taller, even had a few curves, and for the first time I felt confident about how I looked. No more hiding my face behind those big eighties bangs and hair. I also began to earn more scholarship money through beauty contests. Down South, pageants are a cultural phenomenon and offer young women incredible opportunities that they might not otherwise have. I know this is a foreign concept to many of my readers (and, believe me, I've had to defend my pageant experiences to many doubters over the years), but the Miss America system has enabled thousands of girls to go to college and to better themselves and their communities. I first entered my high school pageant as a junior, because I wanted to sing and perform onstage. There was no swimsuit competition; it was just talent and evening gown, and, to my surprise, I won. In every picture of me from that night, my hands are over my mouth and my eyes are as wide as saucers. Once I got into college, I went on to win Miss Gwinnett County and spent many a weekend at ribbon-cutting ceremonies, giving a few speeches here and there, even singing the national anthem. I gave a father-daughter speech at a local church, where my first line was, "My father was never my friend growing up, but I wouldn't have had it any other way." Dad was in the audience, beaming.

My mom did her best to never let it go to my head. She and Dad were always in the audience, cheering me on, and I knew they were proud of my performance, not simply my appearance. But we also had fun picking out evening gowns. It was an incredible bonding experience, and so was having long talks in the car, just the two of us, as she drove me down I-85 to voice lessons.

Of course, there was also the swimsuit competition. The Miss Georgia pageant is part of the Miss America system, and in 1995 they were trying to project a wholesome image, so we were only allowed to wear one-piece swimsuits, barefoot, no high heels. Not incredibly flattering to the legs, so I worked out extra hard. I spent four to five days a week in the gym and pounding the pavement, and I try to stick to that routine to this day.

One thing I loved about Miss America was its commitment to service. Every contestant has a platform or cause. Mine was media literacy—trying to get young people involved politically and socially so they could become better-informed citizens. As much as I wanted to be a journalist, I knew that none of my friends watched the news or read newspapers.

I volunteered at nursing homes from the time I moved to Georgia, but after winning I became even more involved in the community, giving speeches and volunteering at a level I wouldn't have otherwise. I credit the Miss America system for those transformative experiences.

When I was nineteen I met my first serious boyfriend, who ultimately became my husband. I first met Tim when I was working at Rich's department store during Christmas break my freshman year; he was a friend of one of my co-workers. I recognized him immediately when I got back to school. Tim was a big man on campus, very good-looking, and I was a little stunned when he asked me out. He was rush chairman for "Pike"—Pi Kappa Alpha—and he was confident, easygoing, and charismatic. Everybody loved him. I remember jumping up and down and holding hands with my roommate, Ashley, after he left a message for me on my dorm room answering machine.

Tim took me to Taco Bell on our first date, and from that moment on I had a serious case of puppy love. We dated for about four months, and I was head over heels, but I was pretty sure he was just having fun. That was confirmed one night in late April when I was on the phone with him in my dorm room. He seemed distant, so I pushed him about how he felt about *us*.

"Do you want to see other people?" I asked.

"Why does it have to be so black and white? Can't we see each other and see other people, too?" he said.

"No, that's definitely not going to work for me. So is this it?" I asked, devastated.

We broke up, and I cried nearly every night during the summer between freshman and sophomore years. It took me my entire sophomore year to forget about him. It was especially painful for me because

I had lost my virginity to Tim and had been so excited that, after so many years of feeling invisible, someone thought I was beautiful, someone wanted me. Especially someone like Tim.

I would see him across the room every now and then at parties, but we never really talked again until one night right before the summer leading into junior year. Tim was headed off to teach at a boys' camp in Colorado, and at the end of our conversation, which had lasted into the early hours of the morning, he asked if he could send me postcards while he was away. "Sure, why not?" I said. To my surprise, he wrote several letters over that summer, eventually admitting that he missed me. We never talked on the phone—in 1993, no one I knew had a mobile phone. All I had were his letters (which I still have in a shoe box, so my daughters can read them one day). Tim didn't return to Athens until right before fall semester, and when he did, we fell back into boyfriend-girlfriend mode. I felt pride and relief that the guy who just wasn't that into me suddenly was. Once again, he made me feel like I was worth something.

Tim was studying to be a landscape architect, but he wasn't really paying attention to his grades. I helped him write some papers, and he actually went from being on academic probation to making the dean's list. There was never any question about my having a career and making my own way in the world. My senior year, I sent my audition reel around, and I got my first job in Charleston, South Carolina, making $22,000 a year.

I'll never forget the day I was all packed up and ready for the five-hour drive from Snellville to Charleston. This wasn't just going to college; this was truly leaving home. My parents were coming later in the week to help me settle in, but when I woke up at home that morning they were gone. My mom had left a note saying goodbye and that she had to go to work.

So my brother, who hadn't yet gone back to Athens for the fall semester, stood at the front door with his shirt off and a pair of basketball shorts on, waving and yelling, "Bye, sis!"

And that was it. I couldn't believe it. I started crying, and I don't think I pulled myself together until I was somewhere near Columbia, South Carolina. Later, my mom confessed that she was thankful she had to be at work, because she couldn't bear to watch me leave and have that image of me driving away in her head.

As I launched my career a state away, Mom remained hands-down my biggest fan. I sent her all my reporting, to watch on the VCR, and she'd tell me how great it was and every now and then give me suggestions on how to improve. She wanted to see everything I did: every single silly school-board meeting I covered, every crime story I reported.

Tim had stayed behind in Athens. The landscape architecture degree at the University of Georgia is a five-year program, and he had another year to go. But right before I moved to Charleston, he took me to the Biltmore Estate in Asheville, North Carolina, and proposed. I accepted. In fact, I never questioned it. After college, getting a job and getting married were the logical—and expected—next steps.

Tim was such a nice guy. When I told him I was going to have to move around a lot, he said, "It'll be an adventure. Sounds like fun." But then he added a caveat. "As long as we don't have to move to New York."

"Well, that could be a problem," I said, "because that's exactly where I want to end up."

"Okay," he said. "We'll cross that bridge when we come to it."

He visited maybe one weekend a month, making the long drive from Athens. I was nervous about living alone, but I loved my job instantly, and I made such good friends that, six months in, I felt like I had an extended family at WCBD-TV 2 Action News. It was as if I'd known these people my whole life, and I've stayed close to many of them to this day. Newsrooms attract a unique blend of personalities. Newspeople are typically smart, driven, quirky, and flat-out adrenaline junkies. The quirkiness (or craziness) comes with the territory, because if we were normal, we wouldn't do what we do. As soon as I stepped foot into that first newsroom, I felt like I was home. I *belonged*.

Unfortunately, the strain of long distance was starting to show in my relationship. Tim, for all his kindness and good looks, was very different from me, and the distance between us became more and more apparent on each visit. By Christmas, I knew that this relationship wasn't right. It was as if the heartbreak I'd worked through during our year apart destroyed the excitement and energy from my initial infatuation. I would listen to love songs all night long and live vicariously through the lyrics. I watched cheesy movies like *Somewhere in Time* over and over again. I sang along to *The Phantom of the Opera* and *Miss Saigon* and dreamed about a love that intense. I knew that was not the kind of love I shared with Tim. It was nice, it was comfortable, but it was not *song-worthy*. On New Year's Eve we got into a fight that I'm pretty sure I started deliberately, and I gave him back the ring. To be more specific, I took it off and threw it at him. It bounced off his chest, and he turned and walked away. Unfortunately, this happened on one of those quaint little Charleston streets, and the ring fell down between the cobblestones. I felt awful, so I called a couple of my friends, and we spent the next several hours down on our hands and knees until we found it. I felt so guilty, in fact, that I begged for his forgiveness. We got back together.

But after working and being on my own in Charleston, I was beginning to understand what it meant to be young and free. I'd never dated anyone seriously other than Tim, and that spring I met John, the football coach at one of the suburban high schools. He was eight years older than me, really good-looking, and incredibly charming. We met while doing charity work, and then he started to write me letters. Eventually, he called and told me, "The way you're talking, I don't think you should get married. You're too young, and there's too much life to live. You should have that lightning bolt—you should be bowled over. You shouldn't just go through with a wedding because the train's about to leave the station."

He was very persuasive, and eventually he wore me down. Although we never had a physical relationship, we would go to dinner and to the beach, and I felt as if I was emotionally cheating.

Tim continued to visit, and in the early summer we parked his jeep between Sullivan's Island and Isle of Palms—which is right outside Charleston and one of my favorite places in the world—to watch the sun set. I summoned up all my courage. "I haven't cheated on you, but I have feelings for someone else, and I don't think I can marry you," I told him. "It's not right. I don't think I feel the way I should feel."

My heart was pounding; I was being as honest and open as I knew how. I was certain he was going to say, *Fuck you,* get in his car, and drive off, and I'd never see him again.

Instead, he got emotional, which was unusual for him, and said, "Please, give me this weekend to prove to you that I'm the one you should marry."

It was so unexpected and gallant that I lost all my resolve. Stunned, I said, "Okay."

Now I felt even guiltier about trying to break it off, and after Tim headed back to Athens, I called John and told him, "I'm sorry, but I'm going to marry Tim." That was the last I heard from John for several years.

The wedding was set to take place in August 1996, at an antebellum home in Georgia in front of four hundred guests. My mother took care of most of the planning, and as the date approached I started to feel physically sick. Once again, I ignored my intuition, all the while fantasizing about running off to Mexico and becoming a waitress in some border-town café—anything to break away from being cornered and trapped. The night before the ceremony, I completely lost it and, in tears, I told my mom, "I can't go through with this."

Mom was sure I was just suffering from your garden-variety cold feet and had no idea of how serious I was, how long the doubts had been building. "You're walking down that aisle. You can get it annulled later." She was joking, of course, to try to help me through my pre-wedding jitters.

I remember gliding through the ceremony and our honeymoon in a fog of resignation. *Okay, I've made my choice, and I'll find a way to be happy.* We had a beautiful wedding and an incredible European honeymoon, but that made it all the more difficult, because deep down I kept thinking, *Why don't I feel the way a newlywed should feel?* I convinced myself that *I* was the problem. I needed to grow up and realize that the kind of passion I wanted was a Hollywood invention, that I had fooled myself into believing that kind of love existed—but it didn't exist.

And so I carried on, and life was pleasant: I loved my work, and Tim let me have my own life and my own friends. But as I saw friends pair off with that we-can't-keep-our-hands-off-each-other kind of love, I knew I had been right all along. It was possible, and undeniable, and I was jealous. Forget Sunday-afternoon love; I wanted that get-a-room kind of love. I started to come up with excuses. People have always said that I'm not very "touchy-feely." And I thought, *Maybe I don't need a lot of love and affection. I've got a great guy. Good enough is good for me.*

Tim didn't push too hard, and he didn't require much of me other than to just be there. We didn't fight. He wasn't cheating on me. We didn't have money problems. But I didn't feel the way I knew I should about him, and I didn't know how to say it out loud. For all I knew, he felt the same way.

Charleston, with all its beautiful gardens and homes, was an ideal place to be a landscape architect, and Tim got a job with a firm doing exactly what he wanted to do. It's an expensive city, and we didn't have the money to enjoy it much beyond long walks through our favorite neighborhoods and glances through shop windows, but we didn't mind.

Tim's grandmother had left him three thousand dollars when she died, and we used that as the down payment for a house in a quaint town called Mount Pleasant, just on the other side of the Cooper River. The house cost $113,000, which came to $885 a month. It was a cookie-cutter ranch with vinyl siding, but it was ours, and it was brand-new.

At the station, I was on duty for general assignments, but it wasn't long before I became known as the "death and destruction" reporter, because I always seemed to be chasing hurricanes or out in swamps with the cops, looking for dead bodies. Any type of calamity, I was there. These were the days of beepers, and during hurricanes, my mom would convince herself I was being swept off a pier into the Atlantic and would drive me batty with constant pages. True, I was that reporter in the yellow slicker, leaning into the wind, saying, "Yes, it's pretty rough out here, Russ and Nina!" But I was usually careful. I remember one time, between my mom and the news desk, the incessant paging got so bad that I threw my beeper into the woods. (Imagine trying to explain to your boss why you need a new one.)

I love the news business, but it does have its downside, primarily the 24/7 umbilical cord that tethers you to the station. For my first fifteen years on the job, nearly every vacation I ever planned got ruined or cut short—like the time I left Turks and Caicos to go to Detroit in March to interview a serial killer. But you just do it. Some days, you put in twenty hours listening to police scanners, ready to jump into the live truck to race over to whatever is happening. It's also the most satisfying thing I've ever done, other than having my children.

People always ask me how I rose to the top of a fiercely competitive business. There's a very simple answer. I worked my ass off. I did double and triple shifts, willing to follow a story from the morning to the 11 P.M. news. I was always the first one in, last one to leave. I was young and hungry, and able to knock on doors and get people to talk to me.

When you're a cub reporter, you don't have bookers making phone calls for you, and you don't have an advance team of producers. You

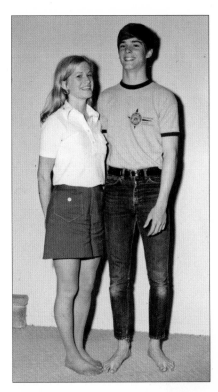

Mom and Dad, high school sweethearts. Benton Harbor, Michigan, 1971.

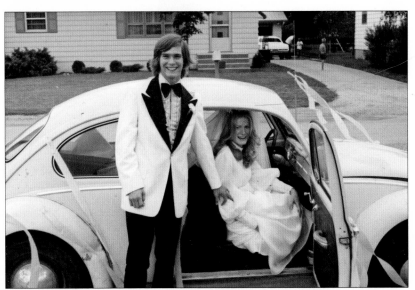

My parents' wedding day, July 1, 1972. They were just eighteen years old!

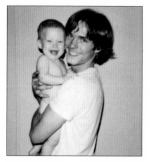

My dad, age nineteen, with me.
Lansing, Michigan, 1973.

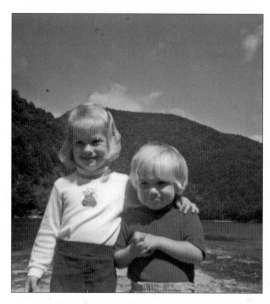

My brother, Eric, and
me hiking with my
parents outside of
Blacksburg, Virginia,
where my dad was a
grad student at Virginia
Tech. September 1976.

Eric and me
on a hot
summer day
in St. Louis,
circa 1980.

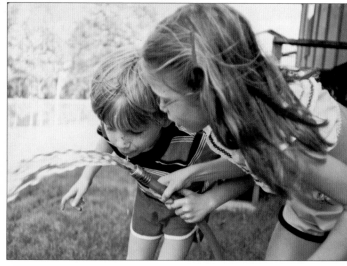

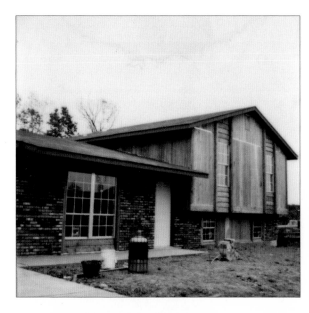

My childhood home in St. Peters, Missouri. I always thought it looked like a smaller version of the *Brady Bunch* house!

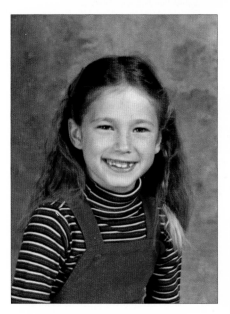

My third-grade school picture. I slept in braids the night before to make my hair curly.

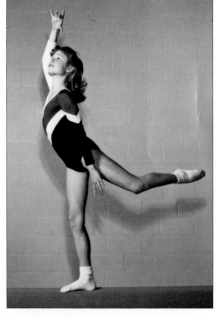

A dorky (and very staged) gymnastics photo from fifth grade, 1983.

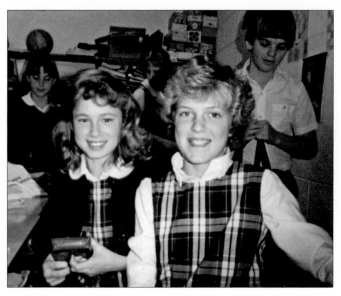

My best friend, Alisa, and me on my last day of school before moving to Georgia. St. Elizabeth Ann Seton, sixth grade, 1984.

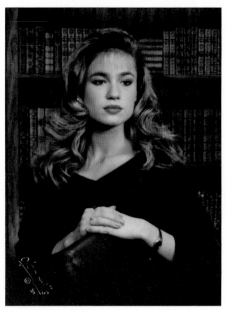

Doing my best to look sophisticated for my senior picture, but oh, man, that hair. Thanks, Rave hairspray. 1991.

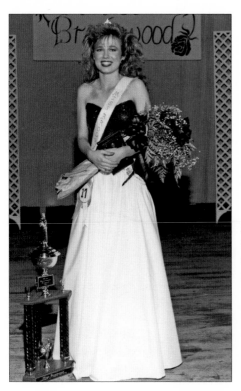

Miss Brookwood 1990, Snellville, Georgia. I was so stunned to win that I had red splotches all over my chest.

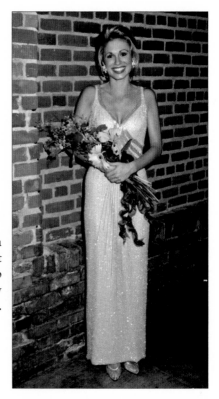

Fourth runner-up to Miss Georgia 1995, Columbus, Georgia. I went straight from the pageant to job interviews, and landed my Charleston job six weeks later.

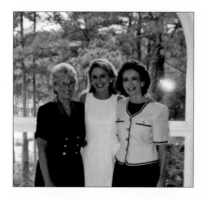

My grandmother (Mom's mom) and my grandma (Dad's mom) at my bridal shower before my wedding to Tim in 1996.

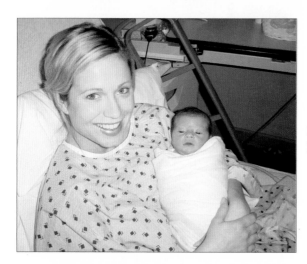

Newborn Ava. December 29, 2002.

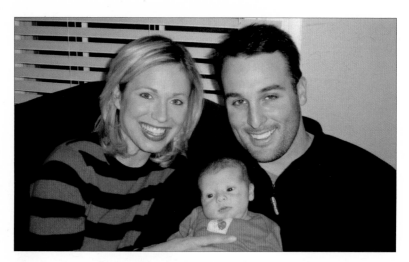

The day Tim and I brought Ava home. My fever started just a few hours after this photo was taken. Washington, D.C., December 31, 2002.

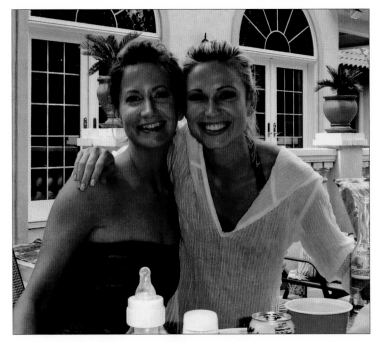

With Aunt Ann at one of my parents' famous pool parties a few months after Annalise was born. Braselton, Georgia, 2006.

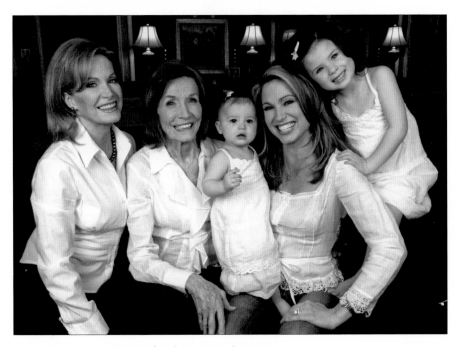

Four generations of girl power! July 2007.

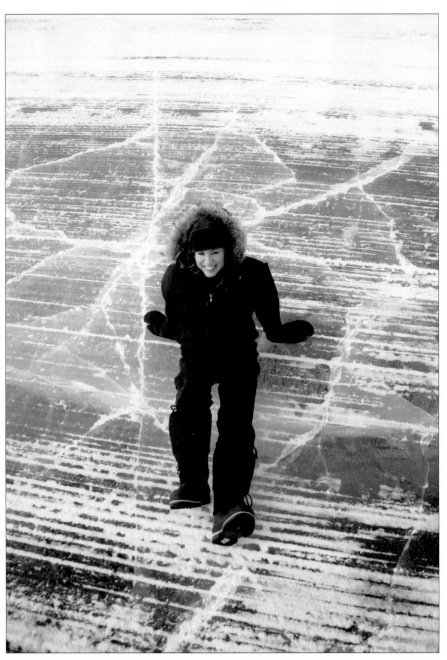

On a frozen lake near the Ice Road in the Arctic Circle, March 2009.

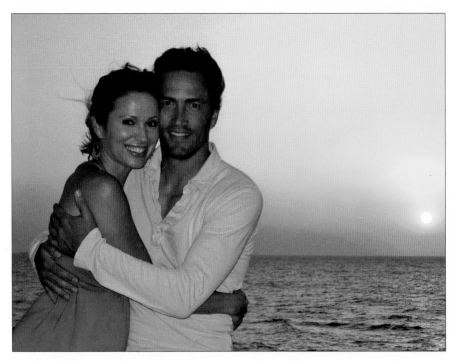

In Santorini, Greece, with Andrew. He "pre-posed" on these cliffs, saying he wanted to spend his life with me. We had been dating for four months. August 2009.

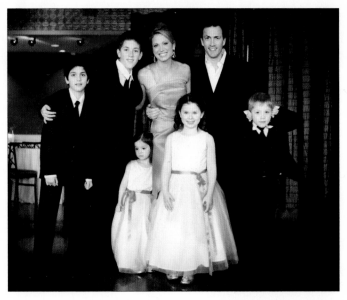

Our new "Shuebach" family on our wedding day, February 6, 2010.

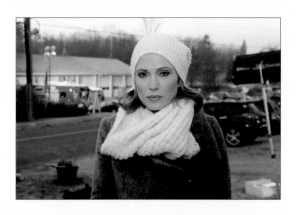

Reporting on the tragic shooting at the Sandy Hook elementary school in Newtown, Connecticut, December 15, 2012. (PHOTO BY ABC/IDA MAE ASTUTE)

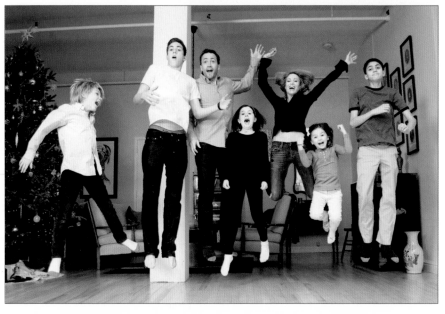

The photo from our New Year's card for 2013, which said, "This is going to be a great year!" Sadly, that wasn't the case.

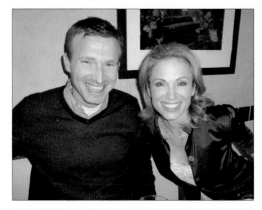

With my brother, Eric, on my fortieth birthday.

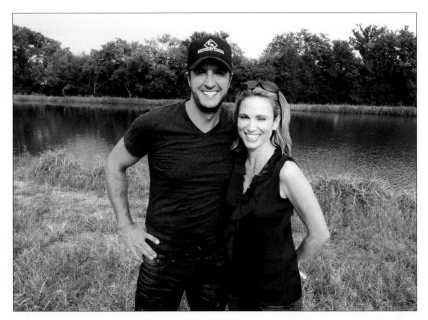

Interviewing country star Luke Bryan at his Nashville farm just weeks before my diagnosis. September 2013.

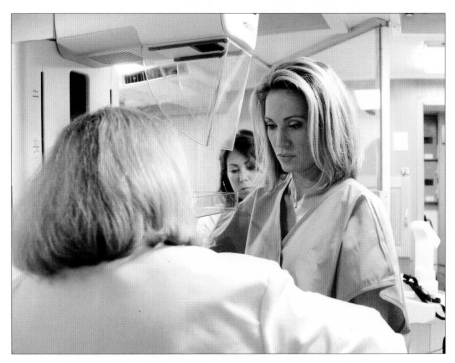

Just moments before my televised mammogram. I was only nervous about how it would *feel* and *look*—I didn't have an ounce of worry about the outcome. October 1, 2013. (PHOTO BY ABC/IDA MAE ASTUTE)

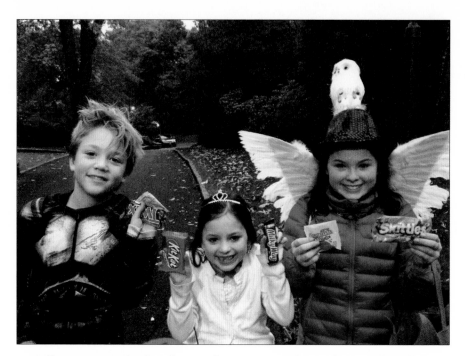

Halloween 2013, the day after my diagnosis. I tried to make everything feel as normal as possible, but later that evening, I had my first of many panic attacks.

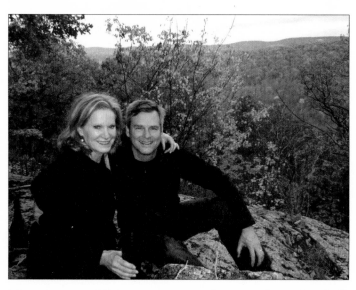

My parents on a hike near our upstate home on the weekend of my diagnosis. November 1, 2013.

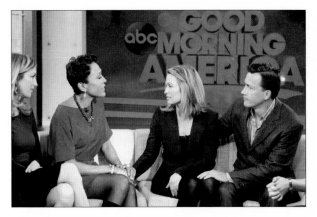

Revealing my breast cancer diagnosis on *Good Morning America*, I was reeling, shocked that the word "cancer" was coming out of my mouth. The moment felt surreal, to put it mildly. November 11, 2013. (PHOTO BY ABC/LOU ROCCO)

The Times Square Jumbotron broadcasting me enjoying the heat at the Winter Olympics while the crew in New York suffered through a snowstorm. (CHRISTOPHER CONATO)

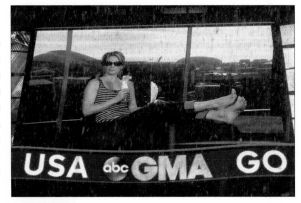

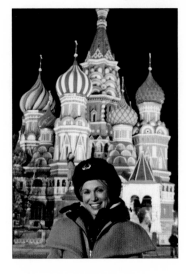

Feeling alive and grateful at St. Basil's Cathedral. Moscow, February 2014.

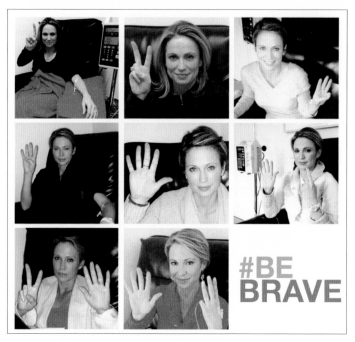

Andrew took photos of me at each round of chemo, and ABC's senior editor of social media, Andrew Springer, created this montage for me with the hashtag #BeBrave. (AMY ROBACH/ANDREW SPRINGER)

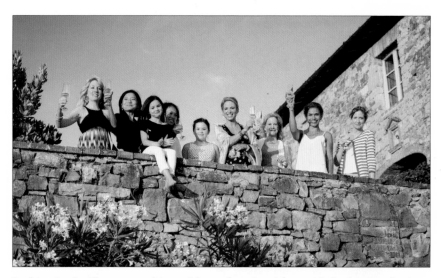

Basking in the Tuscan sunshine with my favorite girls—and the food and wine weren't bad, either! (Jennifer Long, Kaitlyn Folmer, Annalise McIntosh, Melissa Lonner, Ava McIntosh, Amy Robach, Joan Robach, Kristine Johnson, Ann Heibel)

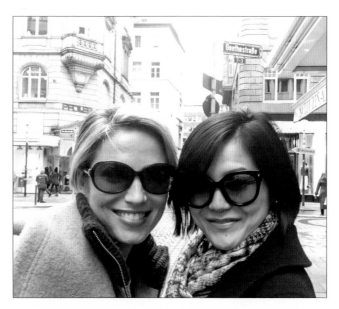

With Kaitlyn in Frankfurt, Germany, on my forty-first birthday (on our way to Sochi). February 2014.

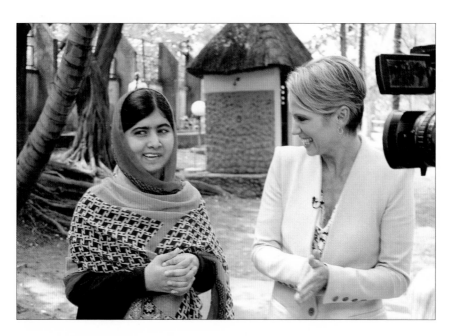

Meeting Malala Yousafzai, one of the most powerful and incredible people I have ever interviewed. Her words and story inspire me every single day. Nigeria, July 2014.

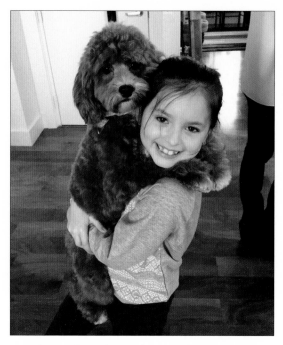

Annalise and Brody. My heart melts every time I see this picture. 2014.

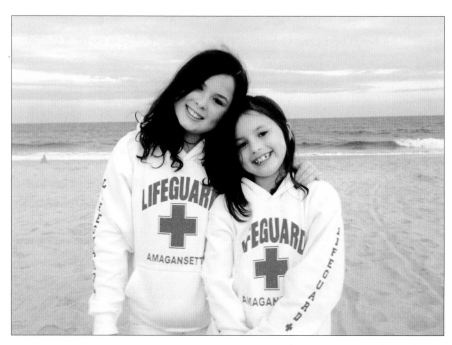

The loves of my life, Ava and Annalise. August 2014.

approach people cold and convince them to open up, when maybe the first thing they want to do is slam the door—or, in South Carolina, wave a shotgun—in your face.

There was always competition with the other stations—and sometimes with my own colleagues—to see who could get there first and then persuade that person not to talk to anyone else. In those days there were three news stations in Charleston, and you didn't want to be the third reporter trying to get the accident victim, or the mother of the shooting victim, to talk. There was a reporter in town who used to joke that his motto was: "Never let the details get in the way of a good story!" I hated when he got there first, because he would ruin it for the rest of us. He'd approach with his cameras rolling and his microphone hot, and if someone came to the door wielding a frying pan, all the better.

But I always thought that kind of ambush journalism was unfair and cheesy. I wanted to engage people respectfully, so I would walk up to the door without a camera. If they were going to talk to me, they were going to talk to me. If I could get there before the other reporters, being polite and compassionate almost always worked. But if the ambush guys got there first, they gave us all a bad name. It feels awful to wait like a vulture for somebody to come out of his house or to try to get an interview with someone who's already told her story three times. But it's part of the job. You have to find the best way to tell the story, even if it's uncomfortable.

My counterparts were mostly men. A lot of the time, I felt that being a woman was actually an advantage, because many of the people we approached at home were women; I could talk to them in a more empathetic way, which shifted the standard dynamic and enhanced the interview. At the end of the day, it's really an issue of trust, so you have to do your best and never give anyone a reason to distrust you. I prided myself on not going for the obvious or the sensational, for trying to find the heart in every story. When people feel something, that emotion becomes the catalyst for change. I want to know more than just what happened. I want to know *why* it happened and, in some cases, to try to stop it from happening again.

I covered some horrific stories. One I'll never forget was about a little boy named Yousef Younis, who went missing during a Mother's Day celebration. Everyone thought he was with someone else, but in fact he'd simply wandered off, alone. There was a creek nearby, and when we went to the house, the parents insisted he would never have gone near the water, because he knew better. We stayed with this family for two days as the search continued.

I was talking to the mother when the police interrupted us. They said, "We need to talk to her."

I took a few steps back and heard them say, "We found your son floating in the creek. We're so sorry, but he's dead."

The horrible guttural sound that came out of her mouth was like an animal being tortured, and she fell to her knees. The pain I felt emanating from her shook me to my core. I still get chills thinking about it.

Those kinds of stories are both gut-wrenching and powerful, because they contain a message. I thought, *Okay, if this is going to be the focus of the story, then what we need to convey is that these are the kinds of things that can happen at parties when no one is being vigilant.* One tragedy can serve as a cautionary tale to help avert more in the future.

Another story that hit me hard was the execution of a man convicted of a triple homicide. In South Carolina, at least at that time, a member of the media had to be present. There was a rotation among the various reporters statewide, and this time I was chosen. I was all of twenty-five years old.

Forty-year-old Sammy Roberts was convicted and sentenced to death for his role in the deaths of Bill Spain, Kenneth Krause, and Louis Cakley, who were moonlighting from Charleston's naval base as gas-station attendants on the night of June 19, 1980. The young men were all robbed, driven to nearby wooded areas, and shot to death. Their bodies were found three days later.

Roberts was arrested later that year along with two other men, Wesley Copeland and Danny Ray Coker. Both Roberts and Copeland were sentenced to death for the crime, after Coker testified against them in exchange for immunity. Copeland died of natural causes on death row in 1986, and on September 25, 1998, I went to the Broad River Correctional Institution to witness Roberts's execution. Once inside the gates, I was shuttled by bus to the Capital Punishment Facility and ushered into what looked like a small, creepy movie theater with a red curtain. No one was allowed to speak; in fact, we had to take a vow of silence out of respect for the somber event. It very quickly became awkward—excruciating, really—as we heard the clanking sounds from behind the curtain as they got everything ready. The convicted killer's pastor was sitting right next to me, and some of the detectives on the case filled the other seats. None of the victims' family members chose to attend.

When they opened the curtain, Roberts was strapped to a table with his arms spread out on metal supports, almost like a crucifixion. When they gave him the lethal injection, his chest shot up and he started gurgling and heaving. The noises he was making were so horrible that the pastor next to me began to hyperventilate and had to be removed. I thought I was going to pass out. I couldn't believe I was sitting there, watching somebody die. I thought I could handle witnessing an execution, that I could detach emotionally, but I was young and unaware of its impact on me.

We sat there for forty-five minutes as he turned blue and prison officials took his vitals to make sure he was dead. There was a phone in the room, in case Governor Beasley called to stay his execution. It never rang. Sammy Roberts was pronounced dead at 6:19 P.M. I signed his death warrant as a witness, and then I went out to give a press conference to about fifty reporters. I was white as a ghost.

When I was in college, and long before the movie *Dead Man Walking* was made, I'd been a huge fan of Sister Helen Prejean, the anti–death penalty activist that Susan Sarandon plays in the film. In one of my speech classes, I even gave a mini-oration against capital punishment. But as a journalist, you don't get to take a stand. When I stepped outside that prison, I found it incredibly difficult to be objective, to tell the story about what happened and not let my personal feelings about the issue cloud my reporting. I did my best to describe what I had seen and to make it clear that this was not a peaceful death. We used part of my press conference in the story for that evening's news. A journalist's job is to give an honest account of what happened and let viewers draw their own conclusions.

All of us at the low end of the totem pole were putting in ninety-hour weeks and making poverty wages. We worked multiple shifts, with very few days off, covering hurricanes, floods, murders, accidents, and court proceedings. It was intense, but we were in it together.

I had a special bond with all of my photographers—we would rotate reporter/photog combos—but I always had my favorites, like Ed, Don, and Kenny. Sometimes we'd have a beer after the show, and we'd talk about what everyone wanted to do in the next couple of years. Some were focused on finding the right person to marry. Others would say, "I'd love to get to Atlanta." Me, I would say, "I want to go to New York," and I'd never even *been* to New York. But I knew I wanted to make it there . . . one day.

Chapter Six

Listening to My Heart

A fter four apprentice years in Charleston, I was lucky enough to get several job offers in late spring of 1999, and one of the most tempting was from KTRK in Phoenix. When I visited, the news directors actually got down on their knees and sang to me in the airport. I knew that if I wanted to work in L.A. one day, that's where I should go, because it was a feeder market to bigger stations on the West Coast. Tim's a golfer, so he loved the idea. And I thought, *I'll finally get to anchor, and the weather is amazing!*

But as I was about to formally accept the job, my agent—whom I'd signed with a year earlier to help me in my job search—called and said, "I just got some interest from WTTG, Fox 5 in D.C. They want to fly you up tomorrow."

I wasn't thrilled. In my mind, D.C. was gritty and grimy, and it certainly didn't have those sunny Arizona skies. Phoenix was the better *position*, as the morning and noon anchor. D.C. would be reporting from the morning helicopter and the noon anchor. But this was the local station where Brian Williams had been the weekend anchor, where Al Roker had risen through the ranks, and where Maury Povich had met Connie Chung.

So I flew to D.C., and they rolled out the red carpet. It was the first time anybody had ever sent a black car with a chauffeur to the airport to pick me up, and I was impressed. After the car dropped me off at the station on Wisconsin Avenue, one of the show's producers picked me up in her convertible and drove me through Georgetown. It was June and I had never been to Washington before. I was blown away by its beauty: the manicured lawns, the lush flowers, the glistening Potomac. We passed the Capitol, the Jefferson Memorial, the Lincoln Memorial, and the Washington Monument, and the power of the city washed over me. I immediately thought, *I'm going to live here.*

I called Tim that night from my hotel room and said, "Don't kill me, but Phoenix is out. I want to take this job—and I know you don't believe me now, but you're going to love this place."

And, Tim being Tim, he said, "Okay, we'll figure it out." That's him: always agreeable, always easygoing.

I was nervous that I was going to be stuck as the "chopper chick," but this was a place where local news was national news, and I knew that given half a chance, I could really grow and prove myself.

The Charleston papers carried the story that I was moving on, and before I left I got a call from John, the football coach who had nearly persuaded me to call off my engagement.

"Can we please have lunch?" he asked. "I just want to talk to you."

I asked Tim first, and his response was, "Fine. I don't have a problem with it. I trust you."

At lunch, John told me he had met somebody. "We missed out," he said. "But I want you to know that I'm happy. And I can honestly be happy for you, if you're happy . . . ?"

I nodded and said, "I'm very happy."

But only because I didn't know any better. And because I still wasn't being honest with myself.

In Washington, Tim moved into construction management, and

one of his first projects was a facility for a government-agency test lab, in which you could safely set an entire building on fire without fear of it spreading. He got to do a lot of cool, innovative stuff, and I was relieved that he had fallen in step with D.C. I felt guilty for making him pick up and leave a city he loved. Guilt motivated me quite a bit in those days (and probably still does in all arenas of my life, especially as a mother). Working at WTTG was as great as I'd hoped, and eventually I got the morning anchor gig as well as the noon spot.

Also, after a year of trying, I finally became pregnant with Ava as I was about to enter the last year of my contract at WTTG. Tim had wanted kids from the moment we got married, but I'd held out for several years because I knew my work hours would never jibe with motherhood. But there came a point where I finally admitted, as my mom put it, that "there's never a perfect time to have a baby," and we went for it. It took a while, but finally, in March of 2002, I peed on a stick, saw those two beautiful lines, and started screaming. I was twenty-nine and incredibly excited, and while I had terrible morning sickness, there were no other issues, so I was expecting a normal delivery.

I worked through Christmas Eve. Four days later, I started having contractions every four minutes, and just before midnight, we went to the hospital. As soon as we arrived, the nurses performed a standard urine test, and I did not have a bladder infection, so they put in a catheter. Upon the advice of my brother ("Don't wait until you feel pain, Amy; get the epidural as soon as you get to the hospital," he'd said), I had my block, and everything was going well.

My girlfriends who'd already had babies had told me how I would feel when it was time to push, because even with the epidural, they said, I'd feel something very specific—an incredible need to make a bowel movement. And when that happened, just six hours later, I called the nurse.

"I'm having this feeling my girlfriends told me about," I said. "They told me this would be when I needed to push."

The nurse replied, "Honey, there's no way you're that far along."

I said, "I'm telling you right now, I'm feeling it, and it's powerful." She checked and, sure enough, I was dilated to ten centimeters.

That nurse rushed to get the doctor, and it was right about then that I started throwing up, nonstop. Another nurse stood next to me, holding a bedpan, and soon I was vomiting blood. I started to get scared. The baby's heart rate was dropping, and everyone looked nervous. My doctor said, "We have to push this baby out *now*."

So the catheter was removed and I pushed, and that's when they realized that the umbilical cord was wrapped around Ava's neck. Every time I vomited and every time I pushed, the cord tightened and her heart rate dropped. They told me to stop pushing. My doctor decided that before heading straight to a C-section, we should try a vacuum extraction, where a vacuum is attached to the baby's head to help guide it through the birth canal. A resident re-catheterized me.

Happily, Ava came out within minutes, and everything returned to normal—for a short while. I spent two nights in Georgetown Hospital in a blissful bubble, resting and feeding her, and then I was released. The very night I got home, I began to feel hot and achy. The next morning, I took my temperature: 103. We were in the middle of a snowstorm, but I was opening the windows to cool myself down.

Eventually I called my brother, who was chief resident at Wake Forest at the time. He advised me to go back to the hospital, but I didn't listen. "That's the last place I want to be," I told him. "I'm just going to pop some Advil." By the next day, I had massive chills and was shaking uncontrollably. My mom and dad had flown in to see Ava, and as soon as they walked in the door, my mom said, "What is *wrong* with you?"

"I'm fine."

"No, you're not," she insisted. "You look terrible."

"It's just a fever," I said. "I think it's my milk coming in."

"It's not your milk coming in! Will you please call your brother?"

"I did," I replied. "He told me I should go back to the hospital."

"Well, then, call the doctor right now!"

This was a Thursday, and when I called the doctor he said, "You probably have the flu."

I said, "I don't think this is the flu. I don't have any other symptoms."

I made the next available appointment, for Monday, and my mom was so mad at me she locked herself in our guest room and started crying. "Please go to the hospital now," she begged me. I kept telling her, "Mom, I'm okay." She screamed at Tim and my dad for not making me go to the emergency room.

By Saturday I had throbbing pain in my lower back. That's when I thought, *Hmm, maybe the hospital isn't such a bad idea.*

And then my phone rang: It was my friend Dianne Risch, who'd been a producer in Charleston with me but had since moved to Chicago. Her family was from the same suburb of Charleston where John coached football.

"I have to tell you something," she said. "I know you'd want to know."

"What?"

"John was killed. He was at a get-together with family and friends in Edisto and was driving home to his wife. He rounded a turn on Johns Island and hit a telephone pole."

The first thing I thought was, *What if I had stayed with him? Maybe this wouldn't have happened.* As I held my newborn baby in my arms, I felt the full weight of his death. He and I had talked for hours about how much he wanted children. He had died on December 31, 2002, the night I brought Ava home from the hospital.

That night, at 2:00 A.M., my mom found me passed out on the stairs. She and Tim scooped me up and drove me back to Georgetown Hospital, while Dad stayed with Ava. I was just conscious enough to be embarrassed by all the drama. I know that no one likes going to the doctor, but I *really* don't. Usually someone has to force me (or, in this case, *carry* me) to the hospital. If my children so much as sneeze, I rush them to the pediatrician, but I always downplay my own health issues and tell myself, *If I wait it out, it will go away.* I don't like people fussing over me. It hinders my independence and makes me feel vulnerable, so I avoid it at all costs.

When we got to the emergency room, they couldn't even get an IV in me, because I was so dehydrated that my veins had collapsed. They had to insert a PICC line—a small hose that ran all the way from my arm to a large vein outside the heart. They did some tests and determined that I had pyelonephritis—a massive kidney infection. They thought it could be traced to when I was re-catheterized before I pushed.

Things went from bad to worse. My blood pressure dropped, and I ended up with lines running into both arms: one PICC line and two IVs. But even with three different antibiotics being pumped into my system, the doctors couldn't stabilize me. My girlfriends were taking shifts with Ava, and Tim and my parents stayed with me at the hospital around the clock. My brother's wife, Michelle, left her one-year-old son, Jack, with her mom and drove from North Carolina to Washington to stay with Ava. Ava was still less than a week old, so it was an around-the-clock job. Needless to say, my sister-in-law is one of the kindest, most selfless people I know. To this day, she and Ava have a special bond, and I believe that week in D.C. had something to do with it.

On day three, when I woke up, my mom had stepped away and Tim was sitting beside me.

I was on a morphine drip, and I could barely talk, but I got out, "Where's Mom?"

"She needed to get some rest," he said.

I couldn't remember ever feeling so weak, as if I might pass out from exertion even though I was lying down. I asked, "Am I dying?"

He didn't respond at first, and then said, "The doctors told us the next twenty-four hours are critical, and then we'll know more."

The big fear was that I'd gone septic, meaning that an overwhelming immune response had flooded my body with chemicals that cause so much inflammation that the organs simply shut down.

Years later, when I got my breast cancer diagnosis, I thought, *I'm going to die from this one day*. But back then, just days after giving birth, I remember thinking, *I'm dying right* now.

For the next couple of days, I was in and out of consciousness, while the doctors continued to pump morphine and antibiotics into me. I should have been getting better, but I wasn't. My parents brought Ava in only once, and I was so weak I could barely hold her.

After another barrage of tests, they told me they had to do exploratory surgery. "Something else is going on, and we don't know what it is," a doctor told me. "It may be placenta that's migrated. Something is causing a secondary infection." They discovered that my appendix was about twenty-four hours from bursting.

I had an appendectomy, and slowly but surely my strength came back. All in all, I was in the hospital for two weeks, but then I had to take a powerful antibiotic, ciprofloxacin, for the next eight months, and a nephrologist monitored my kidneys for a full year.

I went back to work ten weeks after giving birth. I was by no means at full strength, but the war with Iraq had begun, and they needed me reporting from the Pentagon in twelve-hour shifts, from 2:00 A.M. to 2:00 P.M. I put in the long days, and then from 2:30 to 7:30 P.M. I was alone at home, taking care of Ava (we couldn't afford to keep the nanny one extra minute—she was out the door the second I got home from work). Tim often worked late, and I was struggling to keep up my hours, but somehow I managed—until my hair started falling out. I'd lost all my baby weight in the hospital—I called it the IV-fluids diet—but then I inexplicably lost another ten pounds. My doctors eventually discovered that my thyroid had stopped functioning, so they put me on Synthroid, which I have to take for the rest of my life. It all seemed to come back to the infection that entered my body while giving birth.

I joke now that while Ava almost killed me, my second daughter,

Annalise, may have saved my life. When I was pregnant with her—three years later, after we'd moved to New York City—the doctors there noticed that something was off with my blood work, so they scheduled an early ultrasound. The radiologist found a benign tumor called a teratoma, and I was told I'd have to have ultrasounds every three weeks to monitor its growth. Naturally, I called my brother as soon as I left the doctor's office.

"This isn't that unusual, right?" I asked.

Eric started laughing. "It's probably fine, but it's the tumor we all freak out about in med school, because it's so strange and, well, kind of disgusting."

"What? What do you mean? Why?" I asked.

"They're basically DNA gone awry. They can have eyeballs, teeth, and hair."

"Are you kidding me?" I thought he might be teasing me, as brothers tend to do. I mean, this was like a horror movie come to life!

"Not kidding—and can you ask the doctor to save the tumor for you so I can see it, maybe keep it in a glass jar?"

That last part *was* a joke, by the way.

When I got home, I looked it up online. *Teratoma: This is a bizarre tumor, usually benign, in the ovary that typically contains a diversity of tissues including hair, teeth, bone, thyroid, etc. These cysts can cause the ovary to twist (torsion) and imperil its blood supply.*

Eventually, my doctor said I had to have surgery to remove it, because the bigger it grew, the more likely it was to twist. I had surgery two weeks after giving birth to Anna, and even though I felt like I had been to hell and back, I returned to work just six weeks later. I couldn't afford to take any more time off from my new job with NBC and the hefty New York City mortgage hanging over my head, so I rolled up my sleeves and pushed forward.

———

I GOT MY New York job within a few months of returning from maternity leave with Ava. Turns out those twelve-hour shifts at the Pentagon paid off. NBC had taken notice. One afternoon in April 2003, NBC's Olivia Metzger cold-called me at my newsroom desk.

"When's your contract up?" she asked.

I was so shocked that it took me a moment to find my voice. "Actually, this is extremely good timing. In four months," I said.

"Where do you want to work?" she asked. "I place anchors at our affiliates all over the country. Where's your dream place to live?"

"New York!" I said, without skipping a beat. But my heart was pounding. This was the kind of phone call you only dream about. I never imagined it would actually happen.

We arranged a trip for the following week. Sitting in my cubicle at WTTG, I tried to take it all in. I could barely contain my giddiness. My dream was becoming a reality. I loved D.C. and my friends, but I wanted to see how far I could go.

A few days later, Ezra, my agent at the time, got a call from ABC News. After NBC called, Ezra had started sending out my résumé tapes, to see if there was any other interest. ABC was looking for an overnight anchor, so they flew me up before I even met with NBC. I flew to New York twice for interviews at ABC and once for NBC, but I ultimately decided on what I thought was the opportunity of a lifetime: an anchor position on MSNBC.

I was thrilled but dreaded talking to Tim. "I know that you *think* you hate New York, but I warned you this might happen," I told him. "Please don't fight me on this. I need to go." Tim had family in Ridgewood, New Jersey, a beautiful, village-like suburb of New York City. That was our compromise: He could be near family, and I could be near the city. By the time we moved, it was August of 2003 and Ava was eight months old. The commute wasn't terrible, because MSNBC's studios at that time were in Secaucus, New Jersey, a stone's throw across the Hudson River from Manhattan.

The best way to describe my job was news-anchor boot camp. Some people are great reporters but not great anchors, and others are great anchors but don't know how to report. I'd been a reporter my entire career, with a limited amount of anchoring experience, but for the next four and a half years I got an amazing opportunity to sharpen my hosting skills. There were days when I was on air for nine hours without a script, tackling heady stories like the war with Iraq and Saddam Hussein's trial. I managed the art of the live interview daily and learned how to moderate a panel of people who were screaming at one another. (The trick in those situations is to maintain a commanding presence and know when to step in; sometimes you just have to yell *louder*.) When I wasn't anchoring at the cable network, I fought to go out and report for NBC News. I often read the news on *Weekend Today* (giving up my days off), and it paid off four years later, in 2007, when I moved over full-time to the network to become the co-host of Saturday's *Today*. I also got to fill in for Meredith Vieira and Ann Curry—the big guns—and then I would host the nine o'clock hour several days a week. During my years at NBC, I pretty much worked seven days a week.

You might wonder if being "married" to my job didn't destroy my actual marriage, but I'd argue that my ninety-hour workweek *kept* me married. I was so focused on my job that I never had to think about my relationship. I felt lost in the New Jersey suburbs. In D.C., everybody was from somewhere else, but Ridgewood is an incredibly insular community. For the first time in my life, I had trouble making friends. *Maybe if we were in the city, I'd be happier,* I thought. *Too bad there's no way we can afford it.*

And then, right when I was starting to feel totally trapped, something incredible happened: My boss, MSNBC president Rick Kaplan, decided to give me a huge raise. I had interviewed with Rick one year earlier at ABC. He'd since left ABC to try to revitalize the third-ranked cable network, and he had big plans to make it a news destination for viewers: less sensationalism, more journalism. I knew he had liked me when we met at ABC, because at my interview he'd said, "I may not be able to hire you now, but I like you, and—mark my words—one day you will work for me. You have what it takes to make it." Then he gave me a mustard jar off his desk (the closest thing within arm's reach) and said, "Take this home with you. When the day comes that you work for me, I'll expect to get it back." Yes, it was a bit strange but also endearing—and unforgettable.

Sure enough, our paths did cross again, perhaps sooner than either of us anticipated. I had no idea he would be leaving ABC within a matter of months, but I decided on his second day at MSNBC to bring in that mustard jar, and we both had a good laugh. Rick is big in both stature and personality, and he's one of the smartest, most fearless managers I've ever worked for. During his first few months on the job, Rick would make a point to tell me when he liked an interview I did or remark on how well I handled breaking news. You don't get a lot of positive feedback in this industry, and it was especially meaningful coming from him.

"You're a rising star here and over at NBC," he told me, "and you're not making what you deserve. I'm ripping up your contract and doubling your money." All of a sudden, Tim and I could afford that Manhattan home I'd been dreaming of for so many years. We bought an apartment at 30th and Park, and not too long after, I got the *Weekend Today* co-host position. On top of that, I was filling in for Natalie Morales, who was on maternity leave from the weekday show. So I was on the number-one morning show, on the air six days a week. I had achieved every goal I'd set for myself. I had blown away the doubters' expectations of what I could achieve.

Yet I was depressed. I felt hollow and alone. I was constantly worried about what my next story would be and whether it would be good enough. There's a saying among network correspondents that "you're only as good as your last story." I *believed* that. My mood yo-yoed: I would drive myself crazy if I didn't get an assignment I thought I deserved, and when I did get a plum interview, I was on cloud nine—for a little while. Then I would go right back to pacing the newsroom floor, lobbying producers for my next assignment. My self-worth was tied to my job; it defined me beyond the point of healthiness.

Then, as I was in the process of switching from the birth control patch back to the pill, I got pregnant with Annalise. I'd long accepted that with both our crazy schedules, Tim and I shouldn't have a second baby. It had taken me so long to get pregnant with Ava that I never imagined it would happen without any planning! After the initial shock wore off, I was excited to be a mom of a newborn again. It gave me something to focus on besides my career, and when Annalise arrived, I realized that being a mom was the reason I was put on this earth. I felt a pride and a passion for my two girls like nothing else in my life. Annalise was the sweetest baby, and I threw myself into mommyhood and found a way to keep work anxiety at bay for the next year. Ava and Annalise were my life, but eventually I had to be honest with myself. Something was still missing.

In 2008, I began to see a therapist, and I started trying to figure out who I was and how I'd gotten to this place. I finally acknowledged that I'd spent my whole life chasing my dream career, but the more I succeeded, the more my work became my security blanket—something to wrap myself up in so I didn't have to face my problems. There were days I dreaded going home, not because of my children but because of my marriage. Over a period of months, the therapist helped me peel away the layers, and I finally admitted to myself that I didn't have the kind of love I needed in my life. I longed for a powerful, soulful connection with a partner, and she helped me realize that Tim and I *both* deserved those things. I began to accept that, for us, that kind of love just wasn't in the cards.

Tim and I were good friends, and I hope we always will be, but we were never anything close to soul mates. By now he'd become a project manager for a big real estate company, and when he came home he was perfectly content to play golf or watch sports on TV. We had nothing in common. Through my work in therapy, I began to see beyond what was wrong with our relationship and to examine what was wrong with my psychological makeup. Somehow I'd never internalized the message that my feelings mattered and that sometimes you simply can't please the people you love and who love you. I wanted passion and romance. And I didn't want to look back in twenty years and regret not acting when I had a chance to find the love I was looking for. I wanted my daughters to see their mother striving for true happiness. Tim and I both had become so numb it was unbearable. In the critical moments in your life, you have to listen to your heart and look out for yourself. I hadn't ever really done that. Now was the time.

So at the age of thirty-five, for the first time in my life, I did something for *me,* not for my mom, dad, or husband. I did it even though I knew it would upend my entire life and, more painfully, my children's lives. I knew my parents and my brother and my entire family would be extremely upset with me, but I summoned up the courage because I had to keep from dying inside.

I told Tim how I felt, initially avoiding the "D" word. We went to therapy together a few times, but it was so incredibly sad, because I *knew.* We *both* knew. Ultimately, we decided to divorce.

My deeply loving—but deeply Catholic—parents were not at all supportive. My dad told me over the phone, "You're ruining your children's lives." But my strength came from recognizing that if *I* wasn't at peace, my children wouldn't be, either. They needed happy parents, and neither Tim nor I was happy. I appreciate now that my dad and mom were trying to protect me from what lay ahead. They knew this decision would have real and lasting effects on all of our lives, especially my daughters'. They didn't want to see us suffer. Neither did I, but I also knew that the only way up was out.

Tim and I were so young when we met. In the beginning we had lots of fun, but we could just as easily have dated for a semester and gone our separate ways. A deep, intimate connection isn't something you can force. We'd been together for twelve years, but it wasn't as if our marriage needed rekindling. We hadn't felt sparks even when we committed to each other during our junior year of college. We'd been a great team, but a marriage should be based on more than that. And I didn't want my daughters to grow up never knowing what true love looked like.

It pains me to remember it, but when I was explaining this to my girls—in the first really tough conversation I ever had with them—I said, "Have you ever seen Mommy and Daddy hold hands?"

Ava shook her head.

"Have you ever seen Mommy and Daddy hug?"

Ava said no. Annalise was only two at the time and more interested in playing with her blocks.

"Have you ever seen Mommy and Daddy kissing?"

Ava shook her head again, and I said, "Mommies and daddies are supposed to do those things. Your daddy and I like each other so much, and we're very good friends. But we need to find somebody we can do those things with."

Splitting up is always hard, but for the most part Tim and I acted like grown-ups, and we had about as amicable an "uncoupling" as anyone could want. We went to therapy, through mediation, and had weekly meetings for a couple of months, figuring out how to deal with custody and divide everything. I wanted the kids, and he never fought me on it. I got physical custody, and we share custody in terms of parental rights. He sees the girls every other weekend, and we split holidays.

We drew up an agreement and sent it to a single lawyer to file for us. A while later I got a postcard in the mail that said, "You're divorced." The date of our finalized divorce, August 31, was the same as our wedding anniversary. We were married thirteen years to the day. But given the complexities of our arrangement and the reality of New York real estate prices, we were legally separated for quite a while before Tim actually moved out. And during those few months, he showed me what a truly great guy he is.

Neither of us dated at first, but four months later, just after New

Year's, I agreed to have dinner with a man who, unbeknownst to me, had a live-in girlfriend, and a very possessive one at that. She found out who I was, Googled me, and saw that I was married. She started sending me threats, saying she was going to the gossip columns; she found Tim on Facebook, called him up, and said, "Your wife is cheating on you with my boyfriend."

"That's actually my *estranged* wife," he told her. "We're separated, and I'm sure if she'd known about you, she never would have gone out with your boyfriend." He told her about our daughters and convinced her to let the whole thing drop.

So while I was standing there bawling, my soon-to-be ex-husband was defending me. I was so upset that he said, "How about a grilled-cheese sandwich?" He knew that was my ultimate comfort food. I will never forget that act of kindness.

Eventually we sold the apartment, which was a financial disaster because we'd bought in 2005 and sold post-crash, in 2010. As part of our settlement, I absorbed the loss, so I had to write a check for almost $100,000 to the real estate company at closing. My parents loaned me the money, but I was able to pay them back within three months. I've said it before, and I'll never stop: Thank God for my job.

Chapter Seven

Fireworks

On April 7, 2009, I was pulling double duty on *Today* and *Nightly News,* with therapy squeezed in between. It was a long, tough day, both emotionally and physically, and afterward I was supposed to attend a *Today* book party. Two of my producer friends, Mary Ann Zoellner and Alicia Ybarbo, had written a book called *Today's Moms,* a sharp, funny advice book from mothers at *Today* and other walks of life. I had contributed and wanted to help celebrate their first attempt at publishing, but I would have been just as happy to go home, order takeout, and watch television in my pajamas with my daughters.

As I was wrapping up my *Nightly* script, Mary Ann and Alicia appeared at my office door and said, "We're setting you up tonight."

I said, "No way."

"Yes way," they said.

"Who?" I said.

They said, "Andrew Shue." I drew a blank.

"From *Melrose Place,*" they said.

Then I remembered: Billy Campbell. Back in college we used to have *Melrose* parties. Tim and I had even watched the show together. I laughed out loud, because Billy was never my type. I liked Jake.

It was silly, I know. They were just characters on a TV show! I Googled this Andrew Shue guy and learned that he'd been a professional soccer player at the same time that he'd played one on TV. I'd also had no idea his sister was one of my favorite actresses: Elisabeth Shue. I read that he had three sons and had left Hollywood long before to found a digital media company called CafeMom, an online community for moms all over the country. He'd also founded DoSomething.org, a nonprofit dedicated to inspiring and funding young people to take action in their communities through service projects. And, of course, I looked at his picture. He was much cuter than I recalled, and I remember thinking, *He looks even better now than he did back then!* Mary Ann and Alicia told me they had met him to discuss ways his company could help promote their new book, and they'd used me as bait for the party, saying they knew a great girl they were sure he'd want to meet. So even though I wasn't in the mood to meet anyone, I was curious to see if he'd actually turn up.

The party was at an Upper East Side restaurant called Rouge Tomate. Mary Ann and Alicia seemed as excited for me to meet Andrew as they were for their book to be released. We were standing around, speculating about when he might arrive (it felt a lot like high school), when he walked in and right past us. A few minutes later, another producer, Cecilia Fang, literally pushed me across the room and straight at him.

"This is Amy," she said. "She's our weekend anchor and just got back from ice road trucking across the Arctic. . . ." *Enough already,* I thought. *This is officially embarrassing!* And of course everybody was watching, which made it even worse. Somehow we managed some small talk about our children, and then he had to go. I think he stayed about thirty minutes, but before he left, he asked for my number.

"The truth is, I don't get into the city much," he said. "But if I find myself here one afternoon, I'd love to have coffee or something. How could I get in touch with you?"

I gave him my number, picturing the giddy faces of my friends behind me. And there was more excitement to come, because he texted me five minutes after he left the party.

"It's always nice when you don't want a conversation to end," he wrote.

I waited two hours (it's all about the chase, right? I didn't want to seem *too* interested), then texted back. "You seemed normal. You are normal, right?"

He replied by asking me to go for a walk in Central Park the next day. And walk we did—for three hours on a bitterly cold April day. It even snowed, and I remember I was in incredible pain because I'd stupidly shown up straight from work, in four-inch heels. What was I thinking?

For a guy who said he didn't get into the city much (he lived in Princeton, New Jersey), Andrew somehow found himself in the city nearly every day over the next couple of weeks.

"I thought you only came into the city once or twice a month," I said.

He smiled.

We saw each other most days, and if we didn't see each other, we talked on the phone for hours, about everything from how we grew up to where our marriages went wrong to our hopes for the future (after our first awkward meeting, we skipped right past any small talk). But he didn't make any physical advances. For ten days straight—which felt more like ten weeks because it was so intense—he kept planning day dates. We'd go running or walking in the park, maybe out to coffee. Where was the candlelight and wine? Instead, it was all exercise and Gatorade. I kept thinking, *Does this guy want to date me, or does he want a friend?* He did ask me once if I liked kissing. But it was right as we were saying goodbye. I quickly answered, "Yes," and he smiled as he hailed his cab. Still, he was only *talking* about kissing, not actually leaning in.

But then he started writing me poetry. I was with my friend and executive producer Amy Chiaro the night his first "poem on text" came through. He compared me to wildflowers. Amy leaned over my shoulder to read it. "Oh, my gosh, I can't believe it. He's writing you poetry?" I laughed. It was sweet and romantic—and, after all, wasn't that what I wanted?—but it also freaked me out a bit. No one had ever done that for me before, and I felt overwhelmed. I was still in therapy, and one of our big topics was boundaries. I wanted to make sure I was being smart about getting emotionally invested in someone so quickly.

Finally, on April 18, Tim had the kids for the weekend, and Andrew and I went out for an actual date. He picked me up at my apartment and we went to dinner at a charming Italian restaurant in Greenwich Village, Da Silvano, and to a jazz concert. It was incredibly romantic, and I never doubted his intentions again.

But then I got scared. *This is too much,* I thought. *I don't know what to do with this.* I had even texted Andrew, "It would be good if you let me miss you a little." I told my therapist I was going to break it off.

"Why?"

"Because he's coming on too strong. It's just too much."

"Well, how do you feel?"

"I feel like I'm going to throw up. I feel like I can't breathe."

"That's called fear."

"No, it's not. He's too demanding."

"How else would fear manifest itself?" she said. "Fear is physiological. It ties your stomach into knots. Fear makes you feel sick." I'd never thought about it that way. "From everything you've said about him," she went on, "he sounds like a great guy. So why wouldn't you want him to want you? Why would that kind of intense feeling scare you? It sounds to me like you're afraid to love him and to be loved."

The fact is, I simply didn't know how to accept love or handle feeling this intense about another person. Because if you really, truly love someone, you can get hurt. You're not in control; you're exposed. What happens if the person walks out on you—or dies? I had never felt so vulnerable.

Over time, my therapist convinced me to stay with it. "Run toward him instead of running away," she said. "Just do it for another couple of weeks. All those thoughts in your head that you never say out loud—the loving things, the fearful things—say them to him and see what happens. Allow yourself to be vulnerable."

Her advice helped me relax into my feelings, and I grew more confident and open. And then the fireworks went off. Andrew and I became inseparable. We were kissing on street corners, at restaurant tables, in the backs of cabs. My dear friend Jennifer Long, whom I called my "divorce buddy" because she went out with me most weekends when I was lonely, sad, and lost during that period, once sat in a taxi with us, saying, "I'm still here, guys. Can you give it a rest? I'm right here."

On Mother's Day, I told my daughters, "Girls, I want you to meet Andrew." It was also Annalise's third birthday. Andrew came over and I introduced him as "one of Mommy's friends," and he immediately clicked with them. He and Ava ran races down the block and back to our apartment after dinner that evening.

This meeting took place sooner than my ex-husband might have liked, but he had started dating his future wife three weeks before I met Andrew. We had both moved on very quickly, which made me realize how starved we'd each been for love and affection.

In June, I took the girls out to Princeton to meet Andrew's sons. Once again, everything just clicked. Nate was twelve, Aidan was ten, Wyatt was five, Ava was six, and Annalise was three. Aidan wanted to hear all about my job. Nate put Anna on his shoulders and ran around, and Wyatt and Ava became thick as thieves. Andrew and I were blown away. This instant "blending" probably prompted us to get married sooner than we would have otherwise. It felt magical, and we didn't question it.

There were some less transcendent moments, of course. I'll never forget seeing Andrew's house for the first time. He and his sons were clearly used to living a certain way, and their place was on par with most frat houses. There was a Ping-Pong table in the dining room, four reptiles I couldn't name except for the bearded dragon, and—even worse—four snakes, including a boa constrictor. Andrew also had three cats that came in and out as they pleased, and when the sun streamed into the rooms, you could see muddy paw prints on the countertops and coffee table. Laundry was piled up and there was sports equipment everywhere. Instead of curtains, he had tacked up blankets over the windows where sunlight would interrupt television viewing. Only true love could soften that blow. And Andrew did make an effort. I chuckled as I walked from room to room and saw that he had bought candles and lit them in anticipation of our visit. At least his place *smelled* wonderful.

By summer, Andrew and I were both finalizing our divorces, and in August we went on a trip to Santorini, Athens, and Istanbul. My parents didn't like that I had jumped straight into another relationship, and they were especially unhappy that I was vacationing with a man I wasn't married to, but my mom agreed to watch my daughters while I was away.

Those ten days with Andrew were probably the best of my life. We were living a fantasy, with the brilliant sunshine, the sparkling blue Aegean Sea, the hospitable culture, the incredible food and wine, and no children to worry about. I remember thinking, *This is what people write about. This is why people make music. This is why people create art, and write love poems, and kill themselves when it doesn't work out. This is what I've been missing!*

In September, Andrew proposed on a hilltop in Maine, on his father's rural wooded property about thirty miles south of Bangor, in a town called Jackson. We had flown there so Andrew could introduce me to his dad and stepmom, the last family members I had yet to meet. It had all happened so quickly. We decided that before we took the next step, we should meet each other's family members, one by one. I had already met his sister in New York; then we traveled to Atlanta to see my parents and brother, Boston for his brother, and New Hampshire for his mom. Maine was the last stop in our meet-the-family tour. Before we got there, Andrew called and told his dad he was going to propose, and his father said, "How about that—funny you should mention a proposal. I just so happened to find your grandmother's wedding ring in a box in one of my storage trailers last week. I thought about selling it, but something stopped me. This must be why. It's yours if you'd like to have it." Andrew happily accepted.

When we arrived at his father's cabin, we sat and talked for hours with Jim and his wife, Holly. The next day, Andrew said, "Let's take a walk. I want to show you something." We climbed to the top of a hill where you could see for miles and miles. The sky was a bright cobalt blue, the air light and breezy, the sun warm and intoxicating. We were surrounded by lush green mountains spotted with spruce trees and rocky outcroppings. We sat on a birch log to take in the view, and Andrew turned to me and said, "This place means so much to me. We would spend a month here every summer—my brothers, my sister, and me, here alone with my dad—and it was heaven. But then the accident happened, and it was never the same. For the past twenty years, this place has represented sadness and sorrow. I think it's time to bring some joy back to this spot."

Andrew's older brother, Will, was just twenty-six when he fell out of a tree near where we were standing and later died of his injuries. Andrew, his younger brother, John, and his sister, Elisabeth, were there when it happened, and not a day goes by that the three of them don't think of Will and miss him terribly.

Andrew got down on one knee, and I finally figured out what was happening.

"Will you share your life with me?" Andrew asked, and then pulled out his grandmother's ring, a beautiful antique from 1927.

I was shocked. Even though I knew we were headed toward marriage, I never expected it then and there.

"Yes, of course I will!" I said. And then, "Where did you get this ring?"

He told me the story of his father's timely discovery. I swooned. I felt honored. I felt so unbelievably *happy*.

For the next hour, Andrew and I sat there and made plans about where we would live and where we would travel. We knew we wanted a child, and we talked about growing old together. The next day, Andrew and his dad dragged that birch log down the hill, and after his father passed, Andrew drove it to our home upstate. It's sitting in our garage right now, but one day we'll make a beautiful bench out of it.

After I told my parents we were engaged, they made an honest effort to embrace our relationship. They invited all seven of us to Thanksgiving, but Andrew and I slept in separate rooms. Mind you, I was thirty-six, Andrew was forty-two, and we had five kids between us. But her house, her rules. That's the way it always was and always will be. I hear myself repeating similar mantras to my daughters even now.

After Thanksgiving, we started to look at wedding dates. When *Today* producer Cecilia Fang had shoved me across the restaurant to meet Andrew that night in April, she had joked, "When you want me to plan your wedding, let me know." Cecilia had produced the popular "*Today* Throws a Wedding" series for years.

So Andrew and I took Cecilia to lunch and said, "Remember your offer? We'd like to take you up on it."

She immediately started working the phones. Later that day, she found me back at the office and said, "I have the most amazing place: The Lighthouse at Chelsea Piers, sunset. They just had a massive cancelation, so they'll give it to you at a crazy discounted price."

"Sounds great."

"The date's February sixth."

"But that's my birthday!"

"It's the only day they have. They're booked for two years solid. This is the opportunity of a lifetime." *Okay,* I thought. *I guess I'll have an extra-big party on my birthday.*

On Thursday, ten days before the big day, I got a call from Jim Bell, the executive producer of the *Today* show.

"We need you to go to Barbados. Prince Harry is down there for a polo match, and he's sticking around to visit children's hospitals. We want you to have a drink with him Friday night and talk him into an interview on Saturday. You can go live for the show on Monday and we'll fly you back on Tuesday."

Andrew was apoplectic. "You can't do this."

"I have to."

So with our wedding little more than a week away, and the temperature outside at six degrees, I flew down to Barbados for drinks with the prince. *My* prince stayed behind with five kids.

ON OUR BIG day, a nor'easter dumped nearly a foot of snow on New York City and the surrounding area, snarling traffic on the ground and in the air. Friends and family I hadn't seen in years made the voyage to Manhattan in the worst of conditions to our ceremony along the Hudson River (indoors, of course). We tried to keep the number of guests to a bare minimum, and we still had one hundred twenty-five people in attendance—one hundred twenty-five of our *favorite* people. Andrew's mom officiated. We wrote our own vows, and Andrew's son Nate, only thirteen at the time, gave an unforgettable speech about his dad finding love and the four Shue boys looking forward to moving in with the three Robach girls. It was genuine, sweet, and funny, and Andrew couldn't have been prouder.

We had asked our guests to RSVP with their two favorite songs in lieu of wedding gifts. *Voilà,* we had our playlist! At the end of the night, we begged the DJ to stay later than scheduled and got an extra thirty minutes on the dance floor. Still, no one was ready to go to bed, so we invited the remaining partiers up to our honeymoon suite for more drinks and laughter, finally winding down at 3:00 A.M. It was everything I had hoped for.

I WAS IN newlywed bliss until March or April, when I moved back out to New Jersey, in a home we purchased together just outside of Princeton, and my world came crashing down. I was stuck in suburbia again. Suddenly I had *five* children. I was an hour and a half away from work, and more than once I thought, *Oh, my God. What have I done?*

Andrew and I love each other intensely, no doubt. But building a life together is much more complicated than that. When it was just my girls and me, we did what we wanted. We were a unit; we had a rhythm. Now there were five kids to corral. Everything felt beyond my control. Andrew and I have very different parenting styles—in fact, I would go so far as to say we have diametrically opposed parenting styles. Andrew was a very laid-back father, acting more like an older brother to his boys, while I was a fairly strict disciplinarian. And now we were trying to merge the two.

I've never fought with anybody more than I've fought with Andrew. No one teaches you how to become a stepmom or a stepdad, and there is a huge learning curve. Our fights would escalate like the buttons on a blender, from stir to liquefy to crush ice. We were second-timers, with lots of passion and lots of insecurities. We had to focus most of our attention on our kids, who were also learning how to live with one another, rather than on each other, and that was a big source of hurt. I know: The kids should always come first. But when they're not your kids *together,* that can be very difficult to navigate. Ultimately, we always worked it out. That's the test—being able to fight like cats and dogs, because you know that it's safe, that you love each other.

We had a gorgeous house in Hightstown, New Jersey, but the most exciting thing to do there was go to Target (and I love Target, but you can only roam the home-storage aisle so many times before you wonder what else is out there). The commute, a three-hour round-trip drive, was also wearing me down. Eventually, after two years of suburban living, I told Andrew, "I can't do this anymore. I'm a city girl. I can't live in New Jersey."

We decided that Andrew would live half the time in New Jersey with his sons and the other half (when his boys were with their mom) with me in Manhattan. We'd keep the house in Hightstown so the boys could stay at school in Princeton, but we also rented a loft on Prince Street for Ava, Anna, and me. It had three bedrooms and was big enough for the four of us, with bunk beds and trundles so the boys would have a fun place to visit.

Three months after we rented the place, as I was moving back to the city full-time, Andrew's ex told us that she was leaving New Jersey and moving to San Francisco. Our whole plan was upended. Eventually, Andrew agreed that Wyatt could live with her for one year and then head back east to live with us, and Nate and Aidan would go to boarding school about an hour outside the city. For much of the summer of 2012, we all packed into the apartment. It was tight, but it felt like home—until I got cancer, and then nothing felt safe.

THAT SPRING, I was in a constant state of agitation, which got worse in front of the cameras. I thought it was just anxiety, not only because our family logistics were in flux but also because I was worried that NBC wouldn't renew my contract. They weren't responding to my agent, and I was freaking out because I had bills to pay (including that loft I'd rented in the city when I already had a home in New Jersey!).

One day in April, I was reading the news and filling in for Natalie Morales on *Today*. Unbeknownst to NBC, I was going straight from the morning broadcast to ABC, to be interviewed by eight different executives, so even though I'd read the news a million times, I was on edge. When I got to the desk I felt a little winded, as if I couldn't get enough air. Anxiety about my anxiety kicked in, and I knew I was heading toward a full-fledged panic attack. Right before airtime, I signaled Don Nash, who's now the show's executive producer, and said, "Don, I'm freaking out. I don't exactly know why, but I don't think I can go live."

"You can't be serious," he said.

"I've been doing live television for sixteen years," I said, "and I'm telling you something's wrong with me. I feel really weird, and I can't do it." It was 7:58 A.M., and I was supposed to go on at 8:01.

So he said, "Okay, we'll tape it right now and make it look live."

Don saved me with that bit of technical wizardry, but I was humiliated, all the more so when my friend and producer Mary Ann Zoellner said, "I'm taking you to the medical center."

"God, no," I said. "I'm just stressed out."

"Something's *wrong* with you, Amy. You're flushed. Your face is beet red and you're burning up." She grabbed me by the arm and took me up to the medical unit on the seventh floor of 30 Rock. The doctor took one look, gave me an EKG, and told me he'd never seen such irregular heartbeats.

I told him I was kind of in a rush.

He said, "You're not leaving here unless it's in an ambulance. You're going straight to the hospital."

"No way," I said. What I couldn't tell him was that I was supposed to be meeting with the competition in about forty-five minutes. "You don't understand," I said. "I have a series of meetings that I really have to make."

That's when he yelled at me. "HOW WOULD YOU LIKE NOT TO MAKE ANY MEETINGS EVER AGAIN? That's what's going to happen if you die!"

I said, "I've always had a heart murmur."

"This is not a heart murmur."

"Well, I've always had an irregular heartbeat, whatever it is." I was hell-bent on making it to ABC on time.

"This is not an irregularity. This is an electrical storm." He continued to insist that I go to the ER immediately.

I said, "Can't you please just call a cardiologist? I promise you I'll go there this afternoon, but you have to let me leave. I'm late already."

I called my agent, but I didn't want to tell him what was going on, in case he also insisted on medical attention. Instead, I said, "Hey, I have to stay late for some breaking news, so can you tell the guys over at ABC I'm going to be thirty minutes late?"

In the meantime, the NBC doctor was still trying to convince me to go to the hospital, and I told him, "It doesn't have to be that dramatic, I promise you. You can't make me stay if I don't want to."

At which point I called my brother, who listened to my symptoms and concluded, "You're not going to die. You can wait to get to the cardiologist." He called a specialist for me, and I agreed to show up at the office of Dr. Pedro De Armas at two that afternoon.

The NBC doctor was annoyed, but he very sweetly called repeatedly over the next three months to check up on me. (And in the end he was proud that he'd pushed me, because, as it turned out, there really was something seriously wrong.)

I went straight to the most important interview of my life. I met all the ABC executives I work with now: James Goldston, Tom Cibrowski, Ben Sherwood, and Barbara Fedida, among others.

Over the next two hours, I talked to seemingly every person at ABC above the level of intern, but there was no way I could tell them what was going on in the back of my mind—and in my chest. The whole time I was thinking, *They're never going to hire the person with the heart problem.* I work in a competitive business, and to get a job at this level, I had to emit strength—I needed them to see me as a smart, serious, *strong* journalist. I most assuredly didn't want them to think I was weak or sickly in any way. Pretty ironic, in retrospect.

When I went to see Dr. De Armas that afternoon, he wired me up with a Holter monitor, a miniature EKG that you wear in a vest as you go through the day, and when I came back twenty-four hours later he said, "You need surgery."

"You've got to be kidding! Isn't there any alternative, like a pill?" Dr. De Armas shook his head. My heart was in a constant state of bigeminy, which means that every other beat was a misfire. He told me that anything over ten thousand irregular beats in a day means you are likely doing permanent damage to your heart, slowly weakening it. My Holter results showed that I had more than fourteen thousand irregular beats.

"You can wait," he told me. "But without surgery you're going to continue having these symptoms and they're going to get worse, and your heart will eventually be damaged. If you get it now, you can alleviate your symptoms and prevent long-term deterioration. Either way, you're going to have surgery at some point. It's my advice that you have it as soon as possible."

My brother (the first person I called, naturally) was upset. "You don't need this," he said. "This is extreme. This is *crazy*. Have your doctor send me all of your diagnostics. I want to see everything."

Once Eric reviewed my results, though, he changed his mind. "It looks like you have to have ablation surgery," he said. "There's really no other option."

In an ablation, they don't open your chest. They put fiber optics and a laser through the saphenous vein in your leg up into your heart and burn off the parts of your heart that are misfiring. My doctor, Larry Chinitz, told me, "Of all the heart conditions a person can have, you have the one I can cure, so you're lucky."

We scheduled the procedure for a Thursday. That morning I did the *Today* show, which is live, of course, and they asked me if I could stay for the nine o'clock hour. I said I had a doctor's appointment but went ahead and pre-taped something for them.

An hour later at the hospital, Dr. Chinitz walked in just as I popped up on the TV. "Are you kidding me? Are you telling me you went to work this morning?"

"Yeah. Sorry."

"Please tell me you're going to take some time off."

"I took tomorrow off."

"You are insane, Amy. This surgery can take up to eight hours, and you're going to feel terrible for at least the next couple of days. You've got to slow down."

I reluctantly agreed. Luckily, my surgery ended up taking only four hours. I remember hearing the anesthesiologist, who'd seen the results of my Holter monitoring, say as I was going under, "Impressive vest results." That's me. Always striving to be the best.

When I woke up, I felt peaceful for the first time in a very long time. I hadn't realized how these misfires had been affecting me physically— I'd just gotten used to feeling increasingly awful and off-kilter. Before the ablation, Dr. Chinitz told me that as soon as you put some people under, their arrhythmias stop. After the procedure, he told me, "Yours kept going. You went from bigeminy to trigeminy back to bigeminy. But now you're cured. You'll never have this problem again."

I was relieved that he was so confident, and even more so that he was right. Neither of the geminies, bi or tri, has recurred. And thank goodness I had that surgery. If I hadn't, I never would have been cleared for cancer surgery.

On Sunday, two days after the procedure, when I was recuperating on my couch, *Today*'s executive producer, Jim Bell, called. He and Ann Curry were among the few from the show I'd told about my procedure. "I know this is bad timing," he said, "but I need you to go to Illinois today. Someone won the lottery big time."

Andrew was shaking his head and saying, "Really, Amy?"

When I hung up, I told him, "I have to go." I couldn't lift anything, so other passengers helped me get my suitcase in the overhead bin, and off I went.

MAKING THE JUMP between networks can be a tough thing to do. To have a fairly high-profile job at one network and then move to another—many people crash and burn. For a smooth transition, your new colleagues have to accept and support you, and that's a tough tightrope to walk, since there are only a few coveted positions and a large number of people who want them, who've worked their whole lives for a shot at them. But I hadn't been feeling the love at NBC for more than a year. A career in television is very cyclical. You can be flavor of the month one day and yesterday's news the next. You'll never know what you did, what you said, or what happened, but all of a sudden one executive says one thing about you in a room and you're mud. I was on a roll when I was filling in for Brian Williams, Meredith Vieira, and Ann Curry, but then they just stopped asking me. I was the obvious choice when Ann moved to the big chair and Natalie moved to news, because the nine o'clock anchor position opened up. When Savannah Guthrie got it instead, I knew it was time to move on.

I'm the kind of person who's always expecting to get fired anyway. Every time I get an email from one of my bosses that says, "Come see me," I become that Catholic schoolgirl walking up to Sister Patricia, thinking, "What did I do wrong?" and already preparing my apology. There's always someone younger, smarter, prettier, more hardworking, and maybe healthier to replace you.

When I began to feel uneasy at NBC, I started to save money. I had a year and a half left on my contract, and I stripped my life down to the essentials. By the time my contract ended, I had enough money to stay in New York, keep my kids in private school, and live for a full year.

I say "I" because, even after the wedding, Andrew and I kept our finances separate. With Tim, I'd never had my own bank account. This time I made it very clear that things were going to be different, because I didn't want to grow resentful. I knew from the start that one of the major contributors to our health as a couple would be financial independence.

THREE WEEKS AFTER Savannah got the job I'd been hoping for, I did an interview with the "Hiccup Girl," a young Florida woman we'd had on several times because she couldn't stop hiccupping. But now she was being accused of murder, and we landed an exclusive jailhouse interview. Lucky for me, Ben Sherwood, whom I'd met several times at social events and who had just been named president of ABC News, happened to be watching and asked Barbara Fedida to reach out to me. I was in the Tampa airport, waiting to board my plane back to New York, when she called.

"Ben wants to meet with you," Barbara said.

It felt like divine intervention. Hallelujah! Ben, Barbara, and I spent the next several months discussing how I could move over to ABC, what my role would be, and how I could work out the tricky timing. It turned out about as perfect as it could get (if you're someone who doesn't like a vacation between jobs): I left NBC on the Friday before Memorial Day and started at ABC on Tuesday.

Over that weekend, Andrew and I took a quick trip to Charleston to celebrate new beginnings; I also wanted to show him around my old stomping grounds. When you get married later in life, you've already lived a lot, and it's fun to go back and fill in the blanks with your partner.

AT NBC I'D had a distinct anchoring role, but I'd agreed to come to ABC as a general-assignment reporter or "national correspondent." Then, three weeks after I started, Robin Roberts announced that she needed to have a lifesaving bone marrow transplant, and I was called in to sub for her on *GMA*, alternating with Elizabeth Vargas. Not everyone loved me for that. One guy—who, fortunately, was on the way out—said to me, "What's it like to be the new girl and take over the network?" But by and large everyone was very supportive, especially Robin. When Josh Elliott was away, I was the news anchor. When Lara Spencer was off, I did pop news. During alternate weeks, I was out covering stories.

That summer, Wyatt headed out to live with his mom in San Francisco for a year. The older boys would leave for boarding school that fall, and Andrew would live with us full-time in Manhattan. At a time when I was swamped with work and trying to fit in at a new job, Andrew made the transition from raising three boys in the suburbs to being the stepfather of two girls in New York City.

DURING THE FALL of 2012, I covered the presidential election from Virginia and headed to the border of Arizona and Utah to investigate the Fundamentalist Church of Jesus Christ of Latter-Day Saints, Warren Jeffs's polygamous Mormon sect. Several groups of women and children had escaped and were willing to talk about their harrowing ordeal, so we spent more than a week with them, telling their incredible story in an hour of prime-time television called *Breaking Polygamy* on *20/20*.

In mid-December I was filling in for Robin all week, and on Friday, December 14, I headed straight from the *GMA* set to interview a woman about her massive weight problems for a *20/20* piece. That's when Wendy Fisher, who heads up the news desk, called me.

"Drop whatever you're doing and get in your car," she said. "We need you in Connecticut as soon as possible. We're hearing reports that as many as twenty children have been shot and killed in Newtown."

As soon as I heard the words "twenty children . . . shot and killed," I thought I was going to vomit, but I ran out to my car and drove straight there. I would make that commute for the following eight days.

The next day, I found myself in the home of Jessica Rekos, one of the little girls who'd been murdered in her classroom. The beautiful and tidy townhouse was buzzing with activity. Both sets of grandparents had flown up from Florida, and friends of the family were there for support, trying to help the stunned parents cope. Richard and Krista Rekos were a sweet couple, still in their thirties, and dealing with the unthinkable. They had a newborn baby and a little boy, and they agreed to talk to me because they wanted the world to remember their beautiful daughter, Jessica.

I wanted to honor their daughter's memory and make sure they felt comfortable, but I was incredibly nervous, because I knew this was going to be a heartbreaking interview. I couldn't begin to put myself in their shoes. Before we sat down in front of the cameras, I noticed a baby picture of Jessica on the table behind us, and it reminded me of the pictures I have displayed of my own daughters, so I asked, "When was her birthday?"

When Krista said May 10, 2006, I nearly fell over. That was the same day that Annalise was born. Our little girls were both first-graders, exactly the same age. I'd just kissed mine goodbye a few hours earlier, and hers was in a morgue.

I had to leave the room, because I started to hyperventilate. I mean, I really lost it. The reality of what they were living through hit me and knocked the wind out of me. I collected myself in their powder room, and a few moments later we began the interview. Krista talked about the moment she received the call that Sandy Hook Elementary was on lockdown. She rushed in disbelief through the town where she and her husband had both been raised, a place they had always felt safe.

"As I was running, I kept thinking, *I'm coming for you, honey, I'm coming*," she said, choking up.

I cannot recall another time when I worried about the audio on an interview because of my stifled sobs. Listening to the Rekoses talk about the Christmas presents they had already bought Jessica, and how they had slept in her bed the night before, and how they could still smell her in her sheets—it was overwhelming, and I could barely take in their words.

After each day immersed in the tragedy of Newtown, I'd drive an hour and a half home, just to lie in bed with my girls, then get up at two o'clock in the morning to drive back to be live for *GMA*. I needed to be with my daughters on a visceral level, even if it was for only ten minutes as they fell asleep. Then I could get up and do the story again. After Newtown, I hugged my children differently and noticed that I was more patient with them.

On my last day there, President Obama spoke from the White House about gun control, and I was standing by at one of the make-shift memorials, waiting to go live. We'd hired a security team to ac-company us—I thought it was a bit much, but the powers that be wanted to be careful. Apparently, not all the media had been as re-spectful as they should have been, and resentment was brewing among some of the town's residents.

It was a Thursday at two o'clock in the afternoon, and Diane Saw-yer and George Stephanopoulos were about to break in with a special report. They were going to lead with a statement by the president, and then Diane was going to throw me a question about gun control and the mood in Newtown.

As the president wrapped up, a very large man, maybe six four, ap-proached and stood between the camera and me. At first he seemed to be looking at the memorial. I glanced at my producer on my left and then at the security guard, and I heard the director say in my earpiece, "Amy, get him out of your shot."

I looked back over at the man, and I got a queasy feeling that he knew *exactly* what he was doing, how menacing he was being. He began to edge closer, and my heart started to pound, and I knew that something strange was about to happen.

He looked at me and said, "Do you have children?"

I answered, "Yes."

"Then go home to them," he said. "You're not wanted here."

I said, "I'm sorry, sir, I understand that you're upset. But I'm just trying to do my job."

He stared at me intently, a steely look in his eyes. I don't think I've ever been more frightened.

"What network do you work for?" he asked me.

"ABC," I replied.

"Good," he said. "I'll know where to watch tonight." He reached back toward his pocket, and the security guard grabbed him; meanwhile, the director was yelling in my ear, "Amy, Amy . . . We need to come to you in the next thirty seconds. Are you ready?"

"Give me a second. Give me a second," I said.

That's when the security guard came up and whispered in my ear, "He had a hunting knife in his pocket and he was reaching for it." I burst into tears.

The director asked, "Amy, can you do this?"

I said, "Yes," and I pulled myself together and did the live shot. I felt good about it. I noted that people weren't discussing gun control or anything else in Newtown, because right now they were focused on the funeral processions passing by. I said the people of Newtown were burying their children today and tomorrow and that any conversation about policy would just have to wait. This was a period of mourning, and a period of grief, and a period of shock.

When I got off the air I literally collapsed on the ground, pulling my knees to my chest and my hands to my face, and started crying.

I called Kate O'Brian, who was in charge of news operations for ABC, and told her, "I have to go home. I can't be here anymore. I can't do this anymore. I can't do this one more day."

The next evening, I was at Annalise's school Christmas pageant, watching all of the adorable first-graders singing sweet Christmas songs. I sobbed through the whole thing, while all the other parents were drinking wine and laughing. They knew about Newtown, but they hadn't been there. That was a really, really tough Christmas. I was very loving and very grateful, but I didn't feel very joyful.

———

IN THE NEW Year, Andrew's father was diagnosed with stage 4 colon cancer. It came as a complete shock. Jim had all the appearance of a vibrant and healthy man in his mid-seventies, and Andrew and his siblings were devastated. Andrew went up to Maine to bring him to doctor appointments, and when he was in New York he was on the phone for hours each day, talking to his brother and sister, dealing with insurance and trying to schedule second and third opinions. After a few rounds of chemo without an improved prognosis, his father stopped relying on traditional Western medicine. It was devastating, because Andrew just wanted his dad to live as long as possible, but in the end he came to understand that it was his dad's fight, not his.

It was depressing around the apartment, and Andrew and I had already been talking about looking for an escape from the city on the weekends. We had sold our Hightstown house just before Christmas, so we decided to start looking for a house upstate. We spent one Saturday night at a Hudson Valley inn, and when we got home, the super told us, "There's a little leak."

In fact, the entire boiler upstairs had exploded and come crashing down. Our ceiling was hanging, with strips falling off, and everything was underneath twelve inches of water. A third of our property was ruined—our furniture, our bed, our rugs, twenty thousand dollars in damages all told.

Later that week, Andrew had a soccer game. He plays in a New Jersey league with other men his age and is still very aggressive on the field, and he took a knee to his eye while trying to head a ball. He called me from the emergency room and said, "Don't be upset, but I look like Rocky Balboa." He sent me a picture. He was not exaggerating. It was even worse than I imagined. I can admit now that what I should've said to him was: *So sorry, baby, what can I do to help? That must really hurt.*

Instead, I said something along the lines of: *What are you doing, playing like that? This is what happens when forty-five-year-olds act like twenty-five-year-olds.* (This was not my most compassionate hour.)

When my colleagues saw his black eye, the first thing they asked was, "What'd he say?"

"Very funny," I replied.

Now I had an apartment in shambles, a banged-up husband, and my fortieth birthday approaching. On the morning of February 6, 2013, I was filling in for Robin on *GMA,* and the team made a big deal about my big 4-0, surprising me with Andrew and my daughters, who walked a cake onto the set, singing "Happy Birthday." Kaitlyn decorated my dressing room, and it was all very festive. But after the show, my kids went back to school, Andrew went to work, and I went to therapy. In hindsight, it was terribly timed. Andrew and I were working on co-parenting techniques; our therapist wanted to see us individually a few times, and one of my appointments happened to fall on my birthday and our third wedding anniversary. After the emotionally draining session, I wandered out into Union Square. Hungry and alone, I picked out a chicken wrap at the Pret A Manger and started feeling very sorry for myself. *What has my life come to?* I thought.

I called Andrew in tears and said, "You didn't even ask me to go to lunch! I'm sitting here by myself." Yes, I realize I was being unreasonable, but I just couldn't help it.

He immediately left his meeting ten blocks away and came racing over, but I was still frustrated. I said, "It doesn't matter. I've already finished," and started to get up.

He took my hand and said, "Do you want me to make you happy?"

I nodded. "Yes."

"I planned a huge surprise party for this weekend. Your parents are coming, and your brother and Michelle are, too. . . . But now you've made me tell you and spoil the surprise, you dummy."

Andrew had rented out the back half of a dive bar in the Village, but then we had an epic snowstorm (it comes with the territory of a February birthday/anniversary, I suppose) and all the roads were closed, so none of my Connecticut friends could get into the city. Half of *Today* and half of *GMA* showed up, which is a little bit like mixing the Jets and the Sharks, and we ended the evening at Marie's Crisis Café, a gay show-tunes bar in the Village. It's always a good sign when you end the night at Marie's Crisis.

It still took me a few days to get over the hump of turning forty. But I had more immediate issues to deal with. Around that time, Robin began to come back a couple of days a week. She was still physically weak, but she made it work, and I was incredibly happy for her. It was remarkable to see so much strength and courage. Even so, her return threw my role into question. Through the spring I continued to fill in a few days a week and do stories on assignment, but I was not feeling secure.

In May, I was giving a bridal shower for a dear friend of mine, Contessa Brewer, who'd started as an anchor at MSNBC the same day as me. I'd watched her fight through fertility issues for ten years, and now she was pregnant with twins. I was ecstatic. The party was scheduled for Sunday, and I had seventy-five people coming to my apartment.

On Friday, I got a call to tell me that I had to fly to London to interview Beyoncé. "No, no, no. You don't understand. I have to give a baby shower. . . ."

I was told in no uncertain terms, "You'll be flying to London. There's no one else." The show had to go on: There was a big, joyous event at my house, and I wasn't there. I FaceTimed with my friends—there's even a picture of Contessa holding up her phone, with my face beaming in from London and both of us smiling. But I felt awful. It was one of the rare moments in which I questioned why I was living this way and what I was doing in this crazy business.

A few weeks later, Andrew's father passed away, so as the summer began, the mood in our home took a turn for the worse. It had happened so quickly, and Andrew had an incredibly difficult time coming to terms with his father's death, as well as his new living situation. He shut down and became a shadow of his former self. He lost weight, and at times didn't even want to get out of his pajamas. I didn't know what to do or say. I had very little experience with death, and, sadly, Andrew had too much, first losing his brother (and idol) two decades before, and now his father. My job kept me jumping on planes, and I wasn't there as much as I should've been.

In July, I had to return to England to cover the birth of Prince George. I stayed for three weeks, filming a special for *20/20* called *Mysteries of the Castle: Beyond Downton Abbey,* touring the grand houses and the lifestyles of the British aristocracy.

When I got home, I returned to a lot of professional uncertainty. Robin was back full-time that month, and I knew my role would shrink. I wanted to find my niche: I wanted to be the go-to correspondent for breaking news. But by September I was feeling plain old lost.

And that's when Kaitlyn and I drove to Pennsylvania to interview Marie Monville, the Amish shooter's wife. And when I was asked to have a mammogram on the air. And when I got the diagnosis that changed my life forever.

Chapter Eight

"We Need Some Joy"

Thanksgiving came two weeks after my surgery, and I felt immensely lucky to have my girls, my parents, and Andrew gathered in the dining room at our place upstate. My dad made the turkey, my mom made her signature potato dish, and I whipped up my go-to dishes, green bean casserole and pumpkin swirl cheesecake. Andrew built a fire and helped the girls set the table. Before we ate, we took turns saying what we were thankful for.

I said, "I'm just thankful to be here."

My brother called on video chat, which we'd started using regularly. His three boys were in the background, and I heard my nephew James, who was ten at the time, say, "Aunt Amy looks really good." I laughed. I was glad that I didn't look as horrible as he'd been expecting—largely because I knew that a crew of a dozen would be showing up that weekend to photograph me for the cover of *People*.

ON MONDAY, DECEMBER 2, I was back to the drudgery of being a cancer patient. I had a PET scan, which I cried all the way through. The umpteenth IV was shoved into my arm to introduce radioactive material and see if there was any more evidence of cancer. I lay in an isolation room while Christmas music played; the irony wasn't lost on me as I drank a liter of barium while listening to "It's the Most Wonderful Time of the Year." I couldn't have my phone, a book, or even a pen and paper in the room with me, because everything gets contaminated. So there I was, alone with Andy Williams, and then Bing Crosby started up with "White Christmas." I banged on the wall.

"Can someone please change the radio station?" I pleaded. The nurse came in and asked me what I'd rather hear.

"Rap or heavy metal would fit my mood right about now."

"Coming right up."

I'd begun to feel as if I lived in that cancer center. My world had tilted on its axis, and everything had slid out of place. Life around me appeared normal, yet a constant fear of death wouldn't leave me. I felt as if a cloud of doom would hang over my head forever. Sure, there were days when I felt like Superwoman, but they were overshadowed by the times I felt worthless, pitiful, weak, pathetic. I leaned on Andrew and my parents during these moments, some of them more dramatic than others.

Early one morning that December, we were in bed at our home upstate. I was lying there awake while Andrew slept. The sun had just started to rise, and I couldn't turn off the thoughts in my head that were feeding a growing lump in my throat. Finally I surrendered, heaving and crying until Andrew woke up and asked, "What's wrong, sweetie, what happened?"

I had to get it out. I had to say out loud what I had been feeling deep down since the moment of my diagnosis. "I know I am going to die from this," I told Andrew. "I've always had this feeling that I was going to die young, and now I know it's true." Andrew pulled me into his chest and held me tight while his shirt grew damp under my cheek.

"There's no way you could know that, sweetheart," he said. "I understand why you feel that way, but it's just not going to happen. You're going to fight this, and you're going to win."

We lay like that for the next thirty minutes, Andrew rubbing my back and kissing my head while I cried into his shoulder. Eventually I forced myself to get out of bed. Being busy always re-centers me, so I put on my robe and slippers and went downstairs to make waffles. I love making a big breakfast for my family—something I never get to do during the week, when I'm out the door by 4:30 A.M. My parents were already in the kitchen. They'd heard me crying and what I had said. My mom had tears in her eyes. "Amy, I used to think the same thing when I was your age. It's a normal emotion, even without a cancer diagnosis. Please don't worry about that now. You're going to be okay." They gave me a big hug, and I felt like I could face another day. *One day at a time* became my mantra. You can stand anything for one day.

ON DECEMBER 3, I had an appointment with Dr. Smith, the geneticist, and the next day I saw Dr. Oratz, my oncologist. As miserable as I felt walking into the office, Dr. Oratz broke some news that managed to make me feel even worse.

"Once you're done with chemotherapy, I want to put you on tamoxifen," she began. "And, unfortunately, recent testing has shown that in cases like yours it's far more effective for patients to stay on the regimen for ten full years, versus the previously recommended five."

"Ten years?" I said. I had heard horror stories about the side effects, from hot flashes, night sweats, and insomnia to dry skin and swelling fingers, hands, and feet.

"Yes, ten years, Amy. The greatest chance for recurrence with your type of cancer is between years five and ten. I actually believe the tamoxifen will have a larger role in determining whether or not your cancer comes back than the chemo," she said.

Estrogen can fuel the growth of breast cancer cells; tamoxifen blocks the uptake of the hormone. Your estrogen levels go way up if you become pregnant, of course, so Dr. Oratz also told me that, for the next ten years, I should not try to have another child. I was forty. Add this course of treatment and I was out of the reproductive game.

It was a crushing blow. Andrew and I had been fantasizing about a baby from the beginning of our relationship. We had such a powerful connection, emotionally and physically, that there was nothing I wanted more than to have a child with him. A few years before we met, he had undergone a vasectomy, but when we got married he had it reversed, and I went out and bought ovulation kits. I was so excited about the possibilities. I was never one of those women who *love* being pregnant. In fact, I was fairly miserable with Ava and Anna, with morning sickness that lasted until the third trimester, a nightmare given my morning television schedule. But I imagined that *this* pregnancy would be different. I saw myself relishing it from beginning to end, despite the physical discomfort, because it would be my last and because it would be with Andrew.

I told Dr. Oratz that I'd been planning to get pregnant, and with visible relief on her face she said, "Well, thank goodness you didn't succeed. It could've made your situation much, much worse."

If I wanted to even consider having more children, I had about a week to decide whether or not to harvest my eggs and freeze them for potential use by a surrogate. I was so emotionally worn out, though, that I couldn't conjure up the focus necessary to investigate that option. I was dealing with and trying to understand so many other medical issues, it was just too overwhelming. The morning after I got the news, Andrew, my mom, and I were making breakfast, and I started to cry, reeling from the utter loss of control. "I can't believe this is happening—that I'm done, that I can't have another child. I never imagined this would be it for me."

Then my mom said something no one in the room was expecting to hear. "I'll have your baby," she said. "I'll be your surrogate. I'm only sixty, and you did a story about this very situation!" (It's remarkable but true; in Chicago, a sixty-year-old woman had carried her daughter and son-in-law's baby.) "I would do that for you and Andrew," she ended. I was stunned. Both of my mother's pregnancies had been miserable. She threw up all day, every day, for the entire nine months and had to be hospitalized and medicated at various points.

"You're serious, aren't you?" I asked.

"One hundred percent, yes," she said.

I started to laugh through my tears. I was blown away, but I would never put my mother through something like that, ever. "If we didn't already have five kids between us, I might take you up on that, Mom, but as it stands, we'll count the blessings that we have. But thank you. Thank you for just saying that, and for being you," I said, and pulled her into a hug.

Even today, though, I find myself fighting back emotion when I see new mothers with their babies in restaurants, in the park, or on the street. I feel a pang of intense sadness that I will never have a new life inside me again. A few days after Dr. Oratz's news, I was in an elevator, watching a young woman nuzzling her infant. The baby was smiling up at her mama, who was beaming back at her. I wanted to smile, too, but instead I had to stifle an involuntary moan. I know how blessed I am to have two healthy girls, but to not have the option of another baby was devastating.

BEFORE GOING BACK on *GMA*, I'd had a very specific conversation with Dr. Axelrod, discussing how much of my experience I planned to share with viewers. "You don't want to put any extra burdens on yourself right now," she said. "Understand that you will feel pressure to be and feel a certain way, and that you may be judged for your decisions. That won't help you heal, mentally or physically."

I decided to ease into it by visiting the studio the day before I officially returned to work. It was December 4, and I had a good reason:

to say goodbye to Sam Champion, a dear colleague who'd been a *GMA* staple for seventeen years and who was leaving to become managing editor at the Weather Channel. Sam and I had become thick as thieves within a few weeks of my arrival at ABC. That Wednesday was his last day, and I wouldn't have missed it for anything.

I didn't want to distract from his farewell appearance, so I dressed down in jeans and a sweater, didn't do my hair or makeup, and sneaked in to give him a big hug and a kiss. When he saw me walk in, he tried to get me to come out in front of the cameras, but I shook my head and laughed and pointed to my clothes. I was there to support him behind the scenes, and that was it.

It was the first time I had seen all of my colleagues since the mastectomy, and it made me feel *normal* again, something I desperately missed. We popped a bottle of champagne and had a big cake for Sam up in our green room on the second floor. Then a bunch of us went for brunch with Sam and his husband, Rubem, at the Lambs Club, an upscale restaurant near Times Square. For the first time in a long time, I felt hopeful. *I'm here with my friends; I'm having fun; I'm okay. My life isn't over.*

The next day, I went back to work, filling in for Lara Spencer and doing pop news on *GMA*. The rest of the following week, I covered for Robin, and that Thursday I was on *The View,* sitting in for Barbara Walters. I spoke openly about my cancer battle, because *People* magazine had recently released the issue with me on the cover.

Barbara had sent me the most beautiful bouquet of white roses right after my initial diagnosis, and when I ran into her backstage as she was leaving, I said, "Barbara, I just want to tell you how gorgeous those flowers were. They stood out among all the rest."

She said, "You already told me that in an email." Vintage Barbara.

She thanked me for stepping in for her that day on *The View,* and said she was proud of my bravery in coming forward with my story.

In a way, all the publicity—the *People* cover, the newspaper articles, the television coverage—was like a victory lap in a race that hadn't really begun. I had undergone major surgery, but chemo was just around the corner, and I was terrified. Ask anyone: You can pretty much count on me to be the last one out on the dance floor when everyone else has collapsed, and I'll admit there have been many mornings when I've regretted just how late that "last dance" was. Chemotherapy was going to put an end to any revelry, at least for the next six months.

Kaitlyn came up with the idea of throwing me a pre-chemo party. It sounds a little flippant, maybe, but I'm not sure what the alternative was—to go into fetal position and hide under the covers? There was no ignoring the looming, dark unknown, so I went with the fun option. We called it "Amy's Last Hangover."

You can't have any alcohol in your system when you start chemo, so we scheduled the party for four days ahead, on Thursday, December 12. A dozen of my best girlfriends staked out a corner at the Atlantic Grill, a popular seafood restaurant just two blocks from ABC, and Kaitlyn decorated it with flowers and pictures. We laughed, we reminisced, and we had *fun*. In fact, we had so much fun that we were shushed by a group of older women. And this was at a *bar*. In *Manhattan*. So we must have been pretty darn loud.

In those days leading up to round one, I could feel every nerve in my body buzzing. No one knows exactly how you'll react to chemotherapy, and my doctors carefully avoided the specifics of what it would actually feel like, because every patient is different. There's no way to really prepare, so I avoided any research or conversations about it.

December 16 was bitterly cold. Andrew and I got out of the cab on 37th Street, just west of First Avenue, with the winter wind whipping off the East River. We scurried into the building and took an unusually chilly elevator up to the second floor. I know that route so well now, but I can still remember the first time I walked down the depressing brown corridor. With fear and loathing, I opened the door to suite

202—DR. RUTH ORATZ, ONCOLOGY—only to find a wonderful surprise. Sitting quietly in the small and otherwise empty waiting room was Robin Roberts.

I was confused. Actually, I was stunned. *What is Robin doing here?*

She got up, beamed her amazing smile, and we hugged. "I heard you were going to be sitting in my seat today," she said.

Dr. Oratz had been her oncologist, as well, and it turned out that I would be having chemotherapy in the very room, and in the very chair, where Robin had sat seven years prior. "I wanted to be here to walk you down to our room," Robin told me. Once there, she pointed to two oversize armchairs squeezed into the dimly lit space.

"This is where I sat," she said, "and this is where my mama sat."

I began to cry, and Robin hugged me again and told me, "You've got this." Then she left Andrew and me to start our new and scary journey.

I met my nurse oncologist, Beth. She had been administering these treatments for decades, but aside from experience she brought an incredible depth of caring to everything she did. She started out by giving me a powerful anti-nauseant called Emend, which I would continue to take, along with steroids and anti-anxiety pills, for the next three days. And then the needle went in. Dr. Oratz had prescribed a chemo cocktail called CMF, which targets estrogen-related cancers. Beth came into the room every thirty minutes or so to switch out one drug for another.

Kaitlyn had given me a MiFi to enable portable wireless. "You should watch movies and mindless television," she said. "You'll have to stream."

Andrew and I binge-watched *Scandal*, then *House of Cards*. Each chemo session lasted about three and a half hours, with Beth interrupting intermittently. Sometimes when she came in, we'd pause the show and chat with her, but mostly we just watched TV, the cheesier the better, because I felt desperate to escape. Andrew was in that armchair next to me every single time.

Halfway through, Beth brought in cups of ice, which became my least favorite part of these sessions. I had to chew ice for thirty minutes, because one of the drugs caused mouth and throat sores, and the intense cold would keep my now-toxic blood away from the surface of my mouth and throat. I understood the purpose of the ice-chewing, but there came a time when the sight of it could make me dry-heave.

Around hour three, the chemicals were so strong that it was like aversion therapy: Anything with a chemical taste or smell still makes me feel sick. I don't think I can ever drink vodka again, and the next time I see Kevin Spacey, I may throw up, and then I'll be hard-pressed to explain why.

Just when I was thoroughly nauseated, light-headed, and foggy, Beth returned and took out the needle. She gave me a sheet of instructions to take home: how much and when to take the steroid pills, the anti-nauseants, and the anti-anxiety pills, and an injection to give myself the following day to boost my white blood cell count.

When Beth told me about the injection, I assumed it was like an EpiPen, the auto-injector we used when Ava needed epinephrine for her allergies. You hold the spring-loaded needle against your thigh, press a button, and, *voilà,* you've given yourself an injection. But, no, this was a standard, prefilled syringe, the kind that nurses and doctors typically administer. The thought of doing that to myself almost made me pass out.

Beth suggested that either Andrew or my mom do it, but neither one of them was exactly board-certified, so I asked politely, "Can I just come back in tomorrow and have *you* do it?"

She laughed—she thought it was funny that, after everything I'd been through, I was so scared of a little shot—but agreed.

But the shot was far from my only fear. I was nervous about how treatment would affect my body. Right away I started expecting my hair to fall out, though Beth told me it probably wouldn't begin until after about three weeks.

Dr. Oratz had an even more sobering preview for me. "This is something I tell all my chemo patients," she said. "You run the same risk that Robin did of developing bone marrow cancer from the chemo." It only happens in about three percent of cases, but it does happen. This blew me away. It struck me once again how brave Robin had been, and she still is. I couldn't imagine facing more chemo *because of* chemo.

Andrew had a car waiting to take us home, and my parents and girls were there to help me through the next couple of days. There was another surprise waiting back at the apartment: a beautiful bouquet of pink roses—seventeen, to be exact. It's my favorite number and was one of the many connections Andrew and I had when we first met. The number seventeen is significant to him, as well, for reasons I won't get into here, but let's just say it's *our* favorite number now. After every round of chemo, I found seventeen roses, in different colors each time, when I got home.

The holidays were coming, Andrew and I were busy with work and the kids' activities, and I did my best to keep up as if things were normal. But the days after chemo are rough. You are nauseated, forgetful, light-headed, and exhausted. Right as you start to feel better, it's time to head back in for more.

The nausea and physical discomfort are compounded by anxiety, which is compounded by sadness as you feel your vitality draining away. And with all this hanging over your head, it's hard to sleep, especially when you know you have to get up for work at four. So Dr. Oratz prescribed Ativan, because it helps with nausea and anxiety *and* helps you sleep.

Andrew did all the pharmacy runs and, after the girls were in bed, held me at night so I could cry on his shoulder. My mom cooked, helped the kids with their homework, and kept up overall morale. My dad flew in for every round of chemo while juggling his own demanding work schedule—he never missed a session. I had a village of support and love, but things still felt incredibly tenuous. There were already stressors in my marriage, as there are in all relationships, and the added pressure of a cancer diagnosis initially weakened our bond.

This was the opposite of what I had anticipated. I had a vision of cancer bringing husband and wife together in a beautiful embrace of solidarity and comfort. But that's so *not* what happened. I fell apart, and, frankly, so did Andrew. I didn't want him to leave my side. I was needy, and if he had to leave for a few days for work or to be with his sons, I got angry and resentful. On top of that, Andrew had never really emerged from the deep depression he'd fallen into following his father's death. I hadn't known how to fully comfort him then, and now we both felt helpless and scared. We had moments of beautiful love and support but also of distrust and anger. *How could you say that to me, especially now? Why weren't you here today when I needed you?* Here we were, married for only three and a half years, and we'd already faced blending a family, a major move, death, cancer, and then, in the middle of it all, a custody battle.

We were walking out of my first chemo treatment—which Andrew's ex-wife knew—when she called to tell him that she had filed for custody of Wyatt. Within days, Andrew was served papers at our apartment. She took him to court, and he ended up paying tens of thousands of dollars just to prepare for one hearing. In the end, it was decided that Wyatt would live with us during the school year. But in those excruciating months, Andrew had to endure the dual anguish of a wife with cancer and thinking he might lose his son.

All marriages are hard, and the statistics say that second marriages are harder still. Blended families have to navigate different ideas about parenting, ex-wives and -husbands, the emotional baggage left over from earlier failed relationships—and, oh, yes, all the other ordinary issues couples deal with on a daily basis, from who's doing the dishes and grocery shopping to negotiating work trips and in-laws. All those seemingly insignificant fights can slowly chip away at a relationship.

For Andrew and me, our dynamic as a couple had worked like this:

In any crisis, I tended to react more stoically, and Andrew tended to react more emotionally. I was raised to "tough it out," whatever "it" was. But for the first time in my life, I was a vulnerable, emotional wreck. I needed strength and resolve, someone to lean on, and I had expected that Andrew, who is a beautiful and sensitive human being, would suddenly be a solid rock, a superhuman mountain of strength. Instead, there were more than a few moments when we hit rock bottom.

Looking back now, I can see that it was unfair to expect so much from him. We had only been married for three and a half years when all this crap was thrown our way. For dealing with a crisis this existential, that's the equivalent of being on a second date—you're still getting to know each other and just starting to smooth out the kinks.

It was only after we sought help in managing this new reality that we were able to adjust our expectations and find a rhythm that worked. I turned to friends and family for advice, and they all said a variation of: *Give yourself a break. You are going through hell; acknowledge that. It's okay to slow down.* By trying to keep a million balls in the air while fighting for my life, I was putting impossible pressure on myself and on Andrew. I had unrealistic expectations because I was so desperate to keep things exactly as they were. I'd convinced myself that that would make me feel safe and normal. Instead, I felt like a failure, and sometimes I pointed the finger at Andrew for letting me down.

Andrew and I have both been to therapy at various points in our lives, even a few times together, and we've learned how to better communicate our feelings without triggering raw emotion. We try to handle tricky issues and hurt emotions when they arise rather than pushing them down and waiting for them to simmer and explode. (You know, the kind of argument where you're not really arguing about what you're arguing about? When all of a sudden you're bringing up that thing that happened last week and the other thing you wish he'd done the month before?)

I don't want to paint a rose-colored picture of how things are today, either. The demands of both of our jobs are draining, and juggling three kids' schedules in New York City while keeping a watchful eye on, and close communication with, Andrew's teenage sons at school . . . Let's just say it all keeps us very, very busy.

DURING THE HOLIDAY season I was filling in for various members of the team who were away on vacation. Andrew and I had the girls for Thanksgiving, so now it was Tim's turn. He got them on Christmas Eve, and Andrew and I would pick them up early in the afternoon on Christmas Day.

Nothing we could do at home on Christmas Eve would make up for not having the kids with us, so we decided to change the channel entirely. We have close friends, Melissa and Mark, who have a home in Turks and Caicos (for the record, we were friends with them *before* they had a home in Turks and Caicos), and they invited us to spend the days before Christmas with them.

We flew down after the show on Friday, and it was great to simply get out of town, not to mention take a break from winter. I was four days out of chemo, but I still wasn't feeling great, and being in Turks in December was exactly the right kind of therapy. I'm not someone who relishes leisure, but being with my friends on an island with palm trees and sun and surf and heat took my mind off how generally awful I felt.

I read a lot, and I let myself relax, and I even had fun, but I couldn't shake how different this was from any vacation we'd taken before my diagnosis. Only a few months earlier we'd been in Italy with Melissa and Mark, and the year before we were in Scotland with them; on those trips we rarely got back to our rooms before three o'clock in the morning. This was so subdued, I felt as if I'd suddenly aged thirty years.

It was a good time for Andrew and me. We joke that we have three separate lives: one with five kids, one with three kids, and the one we rarely get to experience, when it's just the two of us. I've always maintained hope that our marriage is going to defy the second-marriage odds, because when we are alone, it's always magical. That warm, tingling feeling of love and excitement immediately comes back to me—that same feeling I had during those incredible ten days in Greece and Turkey, when we were madly in love, without a care in the world. It was impossible for me to feel carefree this time around, but Andrew and I were able to reconnect. We held hands. We even managed a slow barefoot jog on the beautiful white-sand beaches. I felt far away from needles and doctors and poison in my veins, and no one wanted anything from me for five days. It was just us, and it was just what we needed.

We flew back on Christmas Day, as planned, but on the way home from JFK our car got a flat tire and we were seriously delayed. It meant we weren't able to pick up the kids and get upstate until very, very late. And we had a big surprise to spring on our gang.

There'd been so much fear and sadness in our home for so long that, in the middle of my *I'm never gonna have another baby* depression, I came up with the idea of getting a puppy. Andrew and I had gone earlier that month to pick him out, but we wanted to keep it a secret from the kids, and the logistics of having him appear in the flesh on Christmas Day were too much. So we'd taken pictures of him, blown them up, and put them in a picture frame. We saved the gift until last; it was nearly midnight when I announced, "And this is a present for all of you."

As they unwrapped it, I could see that they were less than thrilled at receiving a picture frame, and I bit my lip to keep from laughing. But then they saw the snapshot of this adorable apricot-colored Maltese poodle, and we captured them on video, screaming and jumping up and down. They were thrilled but also stunned, because I'd always been the one to say, "You're never getting a dog . . . too messy, too much work." I shrugged and said, "Hey, we need some joy in our life."

I had to co-host *GMA* the next day, but after the show we all met in Westchester to pick up our three pounds of wriggling, tail-waving cuteness. My older daughter has asthma and can't be around most animals, which is awful, because she loves them. I had been told that any poodle mix would be a good bet.

We named him Brody, in honor of our favorite character from Andrew's and my latest binge-watch, *Homeland*. And, just like agent Brody, our little ginger wreaked havoc on our home. (Brody's lucky he's so cute, because he was a peeing, pooping, vomiting mess!) I'd never had a puppy before, and I was clueless about how much is involved with training one. *Oh, so this is why Mom never let me get a dog*, I thought.

Looking back, I will admit that this *may* not have been the best time to house-train a pet, but now that we're on the other side I can say that Brody repaid all the trouble and more in the form of love and laughter. At first he was a welcome distraction, and now he's a member of the family forever.

When I look back now at my schedule at the beginning of 2014, I'm amazed at how much I worked. For someone in the middle of chemo, I'll admit, it was a little crazy.

Just as Beth had predicted, about twenty days in, I realized I had no leg hair. None. I know that might sound great to those of us who have to shave our legs every day, but it was scary. My legs were bare, and my armpits, too—they felt like a bald head, no stubble, no nothing.

I went into work that morning and told Robin. She said, "That's where it starts. Get ready."

Within days, whenever I washed my hair, strands would come off in my fingers. I'd drop them to the shower floor and cry.

When I went in for the second round, on January 7, I asked Beth, "How much and how quickly will it fall out?"

She said, "I wish I could tell you, but everyone is different. On the chemo you're on, some people lose it all, some people keep partial hair. But I can tell you what hair you have left will be brittle, dry, and limp." She thought for a moment, and then she added, "Given that you're on TV, maybe you should think about cutting it."

I'd never had short hair before. I'd already lost my breasts and any hope of having another baby, and now I was losing my hair? So much of my identity as a woman had already been ravaged by the cancer. *I wanted to be the one to determine what I was going to look like.* So this time I decided to deal with it on my own terms.

Laura Bonanni had been cutting my hair since I first came to New York, and she's become a dear friend. As great hairstylists are wont to do, she's stuck with me through the good times and the bad. She helped me with post-pregnancy hair after I gave birth to Annalise, and she helped me through stressed-out hair during my divorce. She even did my wedding hair when I married Andrew, trudging from New Jersey to Manhattan through two feet of snow in a blizzard to be there in time for our sunset vows.

Before I showed up at Laura's salon, I'd captured very little of my cancer experience on camera, but this I wanted to document. I had Kaitlyn and another dear friend and producer, Natasha Singh, discreetly bring in a small DV camera to shoot Laura creating the new me. It was important to have two women I loved and trusted film and produce this part of my story, at a moment when I was feeling particularly vulnerable.

I stayed strong at first, and Laura was kind. She started by cutting just a few inches at a time.

"Why aren't you cutting more?" I asked her. "You're easing me into this?"

Laura smiled and said, "Exactly."

As I watched my hair fall to the floor, I felt the tears building up. I couldn't pretend that life was normal. Then again, it could have been so much worse. Some women have to shave their heads completely, and I tried to remind myself that it might come to that point. But there was no way to know what the next few months would bring, so for now it was one step at a time. *Snip, snip, snip.*

When Laura was done, I hardly recognized the person staring back at me in the mirror. "I look like Justin Bieber," I said.

I knew there would be a lot of reaction, and, boy, was there. Fortunately, it was positive. My colleagues, the viewers, and even people on the street went out of their way to tell me how great it looked. Walking into the studio that next day, I was a new person. I not only looked different, but I felt different, too—like I was geared up for battle—and God knows there would be plenty of fights ahead of me. But I tried to make light of it, joking, "It took cancer for me to find the perfect hairstyle."

Chapter Nine

"This Is Me, Fighting"

The biggest issue at work that January was the prospect of covering the Winter Olympics in Sochi for ABC News. I'd been given this assignment over the summer, long before I knew I had cancer, and I wasn't about to let the disease take it away from me. In fact, one of the first questions I'd asked Dr. Oratz when I was diagnosed was, "Can I still go to Russia for two weeks in February?"

I was surprised by her response: "If you really want to go, and if you'd be horribly disappointed to stay back, then you should go." I'd been working through all the visa requirements and other red tape for months, but one of the corporate requirements for ABC personnel traveling to certain parts of the world is to go through two days of what they call "hazard-duty training." It takes place in Briarcliff Manor, a small town not far from my place upstate. Essentially, they simulate a kidnapping. Trainers put a hood over your head, threaten you, and interrogate you, all to teach you how to handle yourself in a hostage situation. They also take you through an obstacle course as if you were an eighteen-year-old recruit.

I was supposed to start training on January 16, but when I asked

Dr. Oratz, she looked at me as if I was insane. "Amy, you cannot do anything physically strenuous. No one can touch you from the neck down. You've just had massive surgery, and you're still very fragile."

Happily, corporate cut me some slack. "You know what?" they said. "We're going to give Amy a pass on hazard-duty training."

On January 28 I had my third round of chemo, and the next morning I was up at 4:00 A.M. to fill in for Josh Elliott as news anchor. I went in every day for the rest of the week. I also had to do the audio track for the hour-long *Beyond Downton Abbey* special I'd shot in Scotland and England during the summer. Since *20/20* kept changing the script, I kept getting called back, shuttling between Times Square and our 66th Street studios.

And to keep things interesting, Andrew and I had started to look for a new apartment. Our loft was very cool, but it was dark and noisy, being one floor above restaurants and bars, and with all that was going on, it felt depressing. I needed light and quiet.

We found a place pretty quickly, and the final walk-through was scheduled right after my third round of chemo. I went from Dr. Oratz's office straight to the John Street apartment, near the South Street Seaport.

After the apartment manager, Rose, took us through each room, we went down to the kitchen to discuss our move-in date. I was having a difficult time focusing. I couldn't complete my sentences (the words would just disappear), and I could hear myself slurring. I knew how exhausted I must look—my eyelids were at half-mast throughout most of chemo—and that's when I realized Rose was staring at me: *What's wrong with her?*

Reading her thought bubble, I spoke up: "You'll have to forgive me if I'm not making any sense, but I had a round of chemo this afternoon, and I'm a little off."

"Oh, I'm so sorry!" she said. "Don't worry about it at all, it's fine."

But I was embarrassed. The only thing I hate more than feeling weak is other people seeing me that way.

The only way I knew how to combat that feeling was by working. I was departing for Russia in just a few days, and one fact of life about the former "Workers' Paradise" is that you can't trust the blood supply or the medical equipment. We mapped out a plan with a team of doctors and ABC News to medevac me to a hospital in Frankfurt, Germany, should the need arise. I was extremely grateful that ABC was committing so many resources to let me go despite my condition. I would also bring along my own supply of high-powered antibiotics.

I had a compromised immune system and I was in the middle of chemo, so, as you might imagine, my family was not thrilled about my intention to go to what is, medically speaking, a third-world country. A few days before I was set to leave, my parents came back to town for my third round of chemo. That evening, they sat me down and asked to speak with me. It felt very formal, almost like an intervention. They had given Andrew a heads-up, but he stayed out of the conversation, letting them have their say. Mom started crying and begged me not to go. My brother had told them that if I got an infection, I could die if I wasn't swiftly and properly treated.

"Sweetie, this is not a smart decision," my dad said.

"Why are you doing this?" my mom pleaded. "You have nothing to prove."

I started to cry. I said, "Guys, I need you to understand that I'm not doing this for anyone other than *me*. I have to go. This is what I love to do, and I can't let cancer take another thing away from me. Not one more thing." I looked at Mom and Dad through my tears and said, "This is me, fighting. Please don't make me feel guilty about it. If I don't do this, then I'm basically giving in. The cancer won."

Of course, my daughters didn't want me to go, either, which broke my heart, but I also wanted them to see their mom being strong, not crumbling because she was sick.

More than anything else, though, I wanted to prove to myself that I was still me.

On February 5, just eight days after treatment, I flew to Russia armed with a gallon-size Ziploc bag filled with more than a dozen pill bottles. We had a twelve-hour layover in Frankfurt on what happened to be my forty-first birthday. Kaitlyn was with me, and in honor of the occasion she and Andrew had planned a mini-celebration.

She took me to an authentic timber-framed German Bierhaus packed with hearty German lunch-goers, who seemed to be in a festive mood. We were all squeezed into these family-style picnic tables, and everyone was laughing and talking, eating off one another's plates and downing big tankards of German beer. There was sauerkraut and Wiener schnitzel and more varieties of sausage than I could have imagined. What I didn't know was that my husband had arranged for the manager to bring out an apple strudel with candles just as he messaged me to Face-Time him. He had Ava, Annalise, and Wyatt with him, on their way to school, and as we popped up on one another's screens, they started singing "Happy Birthday."

Thanks to the miracle of technology and the thoughtfulness of my husband, it was a moment I will never forget. Meanwhile, the entire restaurant was staring at us as if we were nuts.

Also memorable, but not in a heartwarming way, was our departure from Frankfurt for Sochi. Several bombs had gone off in and around Russia in the lead-up to the Olympics, so, as you might expect, there was rigorous security at the airport.

The gate agent asked in his heavy Russian accent, "You check any bags?"

Kaitlyn and I nodded. "We checked them in New York City," we said.

"You need to pay for them now, before boarding plane."

"We already paid at JFK," we protested.

"You pay, or you do not board."

Then he pointed us in the direction of another airline employee, behind the counter.

"How many bags you have checked?" she asked.

Between the two of us, Kaitlyn and I had checked several pieces of luggage, including a load of camera gear. We handed her our boarding passes with the baggage-claim tags stapled to the back.

"Six bags," she said. "One hundred fifty euro per bag."

We were outraged. This was a shakedown—the most stereotypical welcome to Russia we could have received before even setting foot on Russian soil.

We got her down to charging us for four bags. The bottom line was "no pay, no board," so we forked it over. After showing proof of payment, we were ushered to a second security line. I watched as the Russian airline agent rifled through my bag, pulling out everything I had packed so neatly. When he found my gallon-size bag filled with prescription drugs, he laughed out loud and said, "These all yours?"

I felt the rage flicker inside me, fueled by jet lag and the twelve-hour layover. I was also still feeling the effects of chemo: I was achy, nauseated, and tired, and now I was *pissed*.

I glared at him and said as loudly as possible, "I HAVE CANCER."

That shut him up quickly, and his smug smile faded away. "Oh, sorry," he mumbled, and waved us through. Turns out, pulling the cancer card can be cathartic now and again in the presence of a jerk.

Another three and a half hours later, we were in Russia. I was on the air every day for two weeks. I was still suffering from the side effects of chemo, and the eight-hour time change wasn't helping my stamina. Kaitlyn made me take my temperature twice a day, every day. I had promised my doctors that at any sign of a fever, our medical plan would go into action and I would evacuate to Germany. Three days in, I passed out in a chair between interviews at the International Olympic Committee building. I was weak and delirious, and when Kaitlyn found me, she was concerned I wasn't going to be able to keep up for the full two weeks—but I did. Each day after that, I got a little stronger.

Oddly enough, nearly everyone else in our group got sick, from either food or a virus. But I bathed in antibacterial hand sanitizer and made sure to drink only sparkling water. I even brushed my teeth with it—which is one of my dad's favorite travel tips, along with, "In the shower, close your eyes and your mouth."

My dad the microbiologist has saved me from myself in Malaysia (including the Bornean jungle), China, Honduras, Mexico, and Africa; no matter how much I want that fresh salad or local fruit, I know it's not worth it. I've seen everyone around me drop like flies when they can't resist.

But there were a few hazards I couldn't avoid. They say smell is the most primitive sense, the one most deeply connected with memory, and I concur, because my strongest impression of Russia is the smell of cigarettes and sewage. Yes, I said *sewage*. The city of Sochi was simply not ready for the onslaught of people coming in from all over the world. Perhaps there was a shortage of good plumbers, because nearly every hotel and restaurant I visited smelled like . . . well, raw sewage. Everywhere I looked, workers were feverishly trying to complete projects—nearly finished sod, almost-planted flowers, half-tiled floors; I actually walked down a sidewalk as they were placing the stones in front of me—and my hotel agreed to give me my key only if I promised not to tweet out pictures of the unfinished construction outside my room.

Even worse than the foul bathroom odors, though, was the cigarette smoke. I'd become accustomed to the smoking ban that's been in place for years now in New York and in most European cities, but Russia is a smoker's heaven, with clouds of cancerous vapor filling every venue. After round three of chemo, I was fighting constant low-grade nausea as the chemicals surged through my throat and stomach, and having to breathe in thick smoke from cancer sticks, while fighting cancer, was maddening. I couldn't eat a single meal without a side of cigarette smoke. In a restaurant one night, my dear, dear Russian-speaking producer Dada Jovanovic confronted some of the more aggressive smokers and asked them to go outside. It did not go over well.

So for those two weeks I resigned myself to breathing in what felt like more cancer. I even took to wrapping a scarf around my face to try to limit some of the intake. It wasn't my best look, but it let me feel like I was in control, in however small a way.

Ironically, one of the best parts about being in Russia in February to cover the Winter Olympics was that it was barely winter. I basked in sunshine and sixty-five-degree temperatures along the Black Sea and gazed down at palm trees and beaches from my window. Sitting in my studio on top of one of the tallest buildings overlooking the Olympic Village, I felt like an ant under a magnifying glass. The sun blazed through the windows, heating the room up to the eighties. Sure, there were mountains an hour inland with snow-covered trails, but the athletes complained of treacherous ski runs caused by the unseasonably warm temperatures.

Between our on-air segments, I kept five fans blowing on me, which was even funnier when we saw pictures of the heavy snow falling in New York. We taunted my *GMA* colleagues and their cold weather back home with a shot of me, in a tank top and shades, sipping a tropical drink, my feet up on the desk. They put the image up on the JumboTron in Times Square, where temperatures were in the teens. GREETINGS FROM THE WINTER OLYMPICS!

While it was exciting to be in a foreign country, covering the biggest sporting event in the world, I missed my little girls desperately and questioned my priorities. It was something I had always struggled with as a journalist who frequently travels, but I worried even more so now. Thank God for FaceTime—how did I manage before video chat came along? The girls would call me before dinner—2:00 A.M. in Russia, and the only time we could coordinate a chat. Seeing their smiling faces made me feel like all was right in the world (even if my world smelled awful).

Kaitlyn and I lined up one more adventure before flying home. It had been nearly three weeks since my last round of chemo. The toxins had cleared my system, and I was starting to feel like myself again. We were facing another long layover—this time thirteen hours in Moscow. Although we had been warned that our visas were good only in Sochi, we decided to take the risk and try to get to Red Square. Who knew when we'd get the chance again?

We landed just after midnight, and our hearts were racing as we walked through customs, fully expecting to be stopped and turned around. But we kept right on marching out the front doors as if we were invisible. We got into a cab and drove twenty minutes to the capital.

It was nearly 2:00 A.M. by the time we arrived, but it was worth it to be standing in front of the spectacular, brilliantly colored and iconic St. Basil's. My lungs stung from the frigid air, but I felt totally alive, and it was thrilling. We snapped photos to prove we were there—both of us in the silly Russian tourist hats we'd bought in Sochi—and I even FaceTimed with Andrew to show him what we'd accomplished. At that moment, I forgot I was a cancer patient. As my eyes took in the magical scenery, I realized how incredibly happy and lucky I was to be right where I was.

Chapter Ten

A Trucker and a Pirate

When I got back to New York on February 25, reality was waiting for me in the form of my fourth round of chemo. Before I left for Sochi, I went in once every three weeks—a relatively light chemical load—to minimize the strain on my body so I'd be strong enough to make it to the Olympics and back. But research showed that my treatment was technically more effective if administered every other week. Of course, I was hell-bent on doing it, but Dr. Oratz fought me a bit, concerned that my workload was too much for me to handle the treatment every fourteen days. I insisted that I was strong enough, even promised to dial back on work if necessary.

"I can do it," I pleaded. "I don't want to drag this out."

Once every three weeks would carry me well into June, whereas I could be done by the end of April if we upped the schedule.

"I can handle it," I said. "I promise. If I can't, you'll know." Dr. Oratz monitored my blood cell count every time I came in for chemotherapy. Chemo can lower it, which can lead to an infection, potentially a very serious complication during treatment. "If there's any change, then we'll go back to once every three weeks."

Dr. Oratz finally agreed. I'd have rounds four through eight—my last—every other week. It was one of those be-careful-what-you-wish-for moments, because I immediately felt nervous about what I was taking on. It was impossible to know what my physical reaction would be to this new regimen. But it didn't take long for me to find out.

Round four was really, really tough. The moment Beth put the IV in my arm, the nausea washed over me and my whole body prickled with goose bumps. I'd had a welcome break, and I think that's why this round hit me so hard. The chemicals had cleared and I'd started to feel good again, but I was also exhausted from twenty-four straight hours of travel just days before.

Andrew took a single photo of me during each session, going all the way back to December. I knew I didn't want a video record—that felt too invasive—but I wanted to document what I was going through. I sent each photo to my extended family while I was still in the chair, and they cheered me on in emails and texts. It really, really helped. In each picture, with the needle in my arm, I would hold up a finger (not the one I really wanted to) corresponding to the round. Round four stands out from all the others. My face is puffy with tears, and I look so *angry*. Truth be told, I was. I was jet-lagged out of my mind, and I was being forced to acknowledge that my battle was far from over.

Most of the time, I relied heavily on denial to get me through the day. I would deliberately forget, telling myself, *I'm not focusing on cancer right now. This isn't happening.* But when the IV slid in, I fell apart. That was the one time I *couldn't* forget, and I was so pissed. I did my best to cry it all out in the chemo chair, Andrew there by my side, trying to console me.

And there were other moments where reality hit hard—mostly in the shower. That was one place where I couldn't pretend that I was okay, that everything was normal, because when the water hit my chest, I felt totally numb. All my nerve endings were gone. After the mastectomy, I was in constant pain, but in the weeks and months that passed, it turned into a lack of sensation. I learned how awful it felt to feel *nothing*. The pain was almost better, because it was *something*. As the water streamed down, I would just start sobbing. The benefit of weeping in the shower is that no one can hear you.

During most of the day, though, my attitude was this: When you're going through hell, keep going.

But things got even worse. The day after round four, we *moved*, which, in hindsight, was one of the dumbest things I've ever agreed to do. Maybe I thought it would be a distraction, but it only added stress and trauma to my recovery. I know I was eager to get to our new place farther downtown; I thought a change of scenery would brighten my mood, not only because it gave us more light, but also because it gave us a spare bedroom. Andrew's older boys would have more space when they came home from school, and for the time being my parents had a much more comfortable place to stay. It was a better space for all of us, but the move was so overwhelming, I just gave up.

For the first time in my life, I didn't care if the floor was clean. I didn't care if the boxes were unpacked or the dishes were done. I didn't care if a picture was tilted or hung right. I didn't care that I didn't know where anything was. I didn't *care*. I was too afraid to care anymore. What did all that cleaning, hard work, and organization get me anyway? That low-grade sense of despair and defeat had lingered since the day back in November when I signed my will, but now I let it consume me.

Before all of this, if you looked in my purse on any given day, you would find at least three lists. On Sunday, I write down what I'm going to do hour by hour, each day of the week. Having everything in order makes me feel happy and safe. I've always been comforted knowing what's going to happen next and what I'm going to do next, which is one reason why the instability of living with cancer was so hard for me. All of a sudden I wasn't in control. My lists didn't matter.

After the move, I was so sick and so weak that my mom organized the closets and kitchen and put everything away. Kaitlyn came over that weekend to watch the Oscars, and I could see on her face that she was uncomfortable with how I looked, how the apartment looked. . . . The effects of my condition were too obvious to ignore. She left early that night, afraid she was adding to the stress.

I couldn't quite remember how I'd managed to paint my daughters' room just after the mastectomy. Even when the dog was peeing and pooping everywhere, I said, "Whatever," and went back to lying on the couch watching mindless TV. At the time I refused to admit that I was depressed, but of course I was. My mantra became: *What does it all fucking matter?*

MARCH AND APRIL of 2014 were the hardest months of my life. There's nothing that even comes close to the physical and mental anguish I felt during that time. My fifth round was on March 13, my sixth on March 27, my seventh on April 10. Two days later, my parents, Andrew, and I dropped Ava off at her *Fiddler on the Roof* rehearsal. It was a Saturday morning, and I was so exhausted I felt like I was trying to run through Jell-O. We stopped at a diner to grab some food, and as we sat down, my phone rang. It was my agent, Henry Reisch.

"You're never going to believe the call I just got," he said. "Can you talk?"

"Of course," I said. "What's up?"

"ABC is giving Josh until Sunday at five P.M. to accept their offer," he said. He was referring to ABC's contract negotiations with Josh Elliott. "If things fall through, they want to know if you'd be willing to step into his slot, full-time, effective Monday."

Whoa! This was not what I was expecting at all. Josh was a dear friend, and I didn't want to see him go. But if he got a better deal, and he wanted to take it . . . "You mean permanently?"

"Yep. As in, the promotion of your life."

"Are you joking?" I said. "Of course!"

But exciting as the prospect was, I figured there was only a remote chance that Josh would end up leaving. It was flattering to be considered as his replacement, but that's about as far as I thought it would go. Henry said they'd let us know Sunday night.

This twenty-four-hour period was the only time during my chemo that I was actually thankful not to be completely "there," mentally or physically. A healthy, vibrant me would have gone absolutely insane waiting to know what was going to happen. I would've spent the time running a million different scenarios in my head and driving my family and myself crazy. In the end, I was so out of it on Sunday afternoon that I didn't even have my phone with me. I was sitting on the couch watching March Madness with my dad, rooting for Michigan State. All I remember is that MSU lost.

What does stand out is that I walked into the kitchen and saw that I'd missed a call from ABC News president Ben Sherwood. Of course, I called him back immediately. I assumed he would thank me for keeping the bench warm . . . but tell me Josh and ABC had reached an agreement.

Instead, he said, "Congratulations, Amy. You are the new news anchor of the number-one morning program in the country."

I was stunned, speechless, struggling to compose myself. "That's not what I was expecting you to say," I told him. "Thank you, Ben. I'm in a state of shock, but thank you."

Josh had decided to leave for NBC Sports. In fact, while I was on the phone with Ben, I saw Josh's number on call-waiting. He was calling to congratulate me. Later, I noticed that the email announcing the change had gone out ten minutes before I'd even talked to Ben. I may have been one of the last people to know that I'd been promoted.

I had been completely in outer space. How ironic is that? The person who was always trying to figure out what lay ahead and how to get there got the biggest promotion of her career when her eye was completely off the ball. I was on a million different drugs, and instead of being out networking and glad-handing at dinners, I was home in bed each night by eight. What a remarkable reminder that none of us can actually control what happens. We can only control the grace with which we react.

———

SHORTLY AFTER THE announcement, Josh gave a press conference. During the barrage of questions, he was asked about the woman who would be replacing him at the *GMA* news desk. After some very kind words about me professionally, Josh said, "One of the reasons I love Amy—off camera—is that she's both a trucker and a pirate."

Now, that's not the usual compliment a woman wants to hear, but I know that he meant it in the most endearing way, in part because he is a trucker and a pirate, too. I daresay *a lot* of us journalists are, behind the scenes: truckers because we love the road and will eat anything that's put in front of us (when you're on a job, you never know when you'll get your next meal), and pirates because we love adventure and tend to drink and curse more than is proper. We've scrambled our way up through gritty small-town newsrooms across the country, consorting with cops, lawyers, politicians, and publicists. Journalists are generally well-intended thrill- and truth-seekers. Our jobs are exciting and stressful, and everyone needs a release now and then. So being *down to earth* (my preferred terminology!) is just part of the culture.

But—mostly for the benefit of my mom and my grandmother, who will read this—I feel it's important to note that I didn't start out as a trucker or as a pirate. I was a good girl. I was raised to have manners, to speak when spoken to, and to be thankful for food and other blessings. My mother also taught me that cursing was for people who weren't intelligent enough to have a more nuanced way of expressing themselves. I still believe in all of the above—it's how I raise my daughters—but I do have to admit there's a side of me that embraces the catharsis of the forbidden. And swearing (quietly) came in handy as I walked into those chemo treatments, uttering to myself how much I fucking hated cancer, how much I fucking hated walking into that place, signing in, and heading up to the second floor to watch the poison flow through my bloodstream and rob me of my vibrancy and energy and joy. That's the pirate in me.

———

THE LAST FEW chemo treatments were every other week, and I hadn't missed a single day of work since December, getting up every day at 4:00 A.M. It was grueling, and I had to channel my inner trucker/pirate to get through those days, especially when the weak, scared little girl inside needed all the bravado she could muster.

Thank goodness I had such an incredible work family to help me make it through the broadcast every morning. I wasn't too quick on my feet those weeks, and my *Good Morning America* co-anchors picked up my slack. Ad-libbing, going off script, and reacting to stories and interviews are big parts of the chemistry of the show, and I just wasn't able to add much. I could barely read the prompter some days. Robin was especially understanding. She knew exactly what I was going through, and to see her sitting there on the other side of treatment reminded me that *this, too, shall pass.*

March and April were tough on everyone. Andrew and I had decided to be as honest as possible about what was happening. Initially, the kids had lots of questions about my health, but one of the beautiful things about young children is that they live in the moment, and soon enough I was reminded that *they* are the center of *their* universes. I was grateful that my seven-year-old quickly moved on from questions about cancer to more pressing queries of the day, such as *Who's going to pick me up from school today? Are you coming to my gymnastics practice? Can I have a sleepover with Jaya and Quinn?*

I was struck by how Ava, only three and a half years older than her sister, had a more empathetic take. She was old enough to feel the weight of my diagnosis and worried about me constantly, always asking how I was feeling, while struggling with her own fear. I consciously decided to inject "cancer humor" into conversations as much as possible. It was my way of making that loaded, scary word less frightening.

One evening, toward the end of my chemo treatments, Ava was

complaining about a skin reaction to some lotion. "Mom," she said, "why do I have to have such sensitive skin? It's not fair!"

I responded in my best whiny tween voice: "I don't know, Ava. Why do I have to have cancer? It's not fair!"

She laughed out loud. "Fair enough, Mom. But you can only pull the cancer card for a little while longer!" That's when we both laughed.

Truth be told, the mood in the house was all too often morose. We were all frightened, and I was so tired that many days I was not at my best. Those were the times I felt guilty for bringing everybody down.

My mother is a hard worker, and a fighter, but—like most moms—she's also a worrier. Toward the end of my chemo, she simply broke down. She started having heart arrhythmias. She stopped eating, and she even started losing her hair. A different reality set in. The scariest part of the journey was the question mark that came afterward—and that's the part that began to wear her down.

The only positive to this time, when my mom needed a little help, is that it allowed me to bond more closely with my dad. He's always been a tough guy who doesn't show a lot of emotion. When I was growing up, he traveled so much that there weren't many quiet moments for us together. But during this period, when Mom and I were both reeling, he truly came through, and I felt the full force of his love buoying me up.

My grandmother, who was also deeply affected by my illness, was another source of strength and determination for me. At eighty-eight, she was not in great health, yet she refused to go to a nursing home, and if there was any way she could work it out, she was also refusing to die! "Amy," she told me on the phone one afternoon, "I'm not ready to go. I don't want to die. I'm not saying I'm not a religious person, but I want to stay here with my children."

THE DAY I'D been waiting for since just before Thanksgiving, when I found out I'd undergo eight rounds of chemotherapy, finally arrived.

Thursday, April 24, at two-thirty, was my last treatment, which meant that *I'd made it*. So why did I feel nervous and overwhelmed with emotion?

I got up at 4:00 A.M. and went to work, as I had every morning since becoming *GMA*'s news anchor nearly a month before, but today I could feel butterflies in my stomach, and it wasn't just excitement. It was fear.

As I dug deeper into why I was feeling so much anxiety when I'd expected to feel relief, I realized that it was because I didn't know where I was headed after today. Everything until now had been charted out—which I always prefer, even when the road map sucks. I'd been on a schedule for battling cancer, and now it was over. And then a question rose to the surface that had been lurking in the background all along: *Will this be my last round of chemo* ever? The answer, of course, was that there *was* no answer. I didn't want to feel too happy and relieved, because I didn't want to get my hopes up when they could be shattered in another six months, or five years. The truth was, I didn't really know how to feel.

When I got to the set that morning, Robin said, "I hear today's your last round. Congratulations."

I smiled and thanked her. But I'm sure she could see my trepidation, because she read back to me what must have been written all over my face.

"Sometimes the hardest part is when the treatment is over," she said. "You feel like you're not doing anything to fight anymore."

I nodded and laughed nervously.

"Your body will be exhausted, and you may battle some depression," she went on. "Talk to Dr. Oratz. You need to know what to expect, and it's not what most people think. I know it wasn't for me."

Then she paused. "But today is a day to celebrate."

She mentioned something about a "small bubble party," which I didn't think much of, as I was counting down the hours until my appointment.

———

As ANDREW AND I pulled up to Dr. Oratz's building on 37th Street, I found myself taking in all the sights and smells as I never had before. It was so much warmer out than it had been back in December, and as I breathed in the fresh air I could feel a kind of awakening in me, as well. We signed in with the doorman for what I hoped was the last time, then rode up in the elevator and went in to face the big number eight.

Andrew and I held hands as we walked into the waiting room. The receptionists greeted us with "You made it! This is it!"

I smiled, and the tears weren't far behind.

As my nurse, Beth, came in, she exclaimed, "It's your last treatment!" and gave me a big hug.

She wrapped the tourniquet around my arm and readied the IV, and Andrew got out his iPhone. He wanted to document my last round, and he started asking me how I felt and what my hopes were for the future. I told him that everything for me, everything I was fighting for, was about my daughters.

I could no longer tolerate ice cubes, so I'd brought in some fruit Popsicles. (Now, of course, I can no longer eat ice *or* Popsicles—just the smell of a pineapple Popsicle sets my gag reflex in motion.)

The room was dark and windowless, and we turned off the overhead lights, leaving on only the small lamp in the corner. Even though I hated coming here, it was my cocoon, the place I'd battled this disease—and my own demons—in the most direct way.

The time went by in a haze. Then it was time to eat the Popsicles, and I knew I had only about forty-five minutes left. That's when my producer Natasha Singh knocked on the door. Natasha had shot and produced my haircut piece for *GMA,* which was the last cancer story I'd shared on the show. She was a good friend and a brilliant producer. I trusted her implicitly with such an intimate and personal moment. She walked in carrying an unobtrusive camera. I had decided, here in round eight, to pull back the curtains and let our viewers in.

With the IV still in my arm, I looked to the camera and said, "Today marks my eighth round of chemo. This is my final round of treatment. The doctors say I 'graduate' today. I decided to have most of my medical moments remain private, but this one I wanted to share. This is a huge milestone for me and for anyone else who has battled cancer. And I join the ranks of 2.8 million U.S. women who are breast cancer survivors. I plan on living each day to the very fullest, thankful and grateful, and encouraging so many women out there who are still in the thick of it, who have yet to fight this fight, that you can do it, you can get through this, one step at a time. And I am there for you. I am there with you." The whole thing took less than ten minutes. Eventually, the IV bag dripped its last bit of poison, the machine beeped, and Beth came back in. Only this time she was holding a bottle of children's bubbles.

She told me Dr. Oratz wanted to talk to me about the days, weeks, and months ahead. "But first," she said, "let's celebrate!" She opened the bottle, took out the small plastic wand, and blew a cloud of bubbles all over me. "As these bubbles reach you," she said, "may they bring you happiness and health."

Andrew captured it all on his phone, a truly beautiful moment that ended with a big hug and, again, tears—but this time, finally, tears of joy. I was light-headed, dizzy, and nauseated, but I was done.

Beth handed me a prescription, written on Dr. Oratz's familiar Rx paper, but in Beth's handwriting. I was confused. I had the procedure down by now, and I'd already picked up all my drugs for this last round.

Beth explained, "You'll feel far too awful to properly celebrate this milestone tonight, Amy. So here's a prescription for you. You need to fill it two Thursdays from now."

I looked at the note. It said, "Celebrate May 8!"

Beth continued, "That would be the next time you'd come in for chemo if you were still in treatment. So that's when I want you to celebrate, because you won't be headed here!"

Next, Dr. Oratz came in and told me, "I know you're going to expect to feel better each day, but that's not how it usually goes. You'll have bad days, and then a better day, and then you'll feel awful again. It ebbs and flows." She paused for a moment, then added, "Remember, you have a lot of chemicals in your body, and they'll still be there weeks or even months from now. So give yourself a break, Amy. You've been through hell."

My breast reconstruction surgery was coming up in early June, and we scheduled an appointment for later in the month to get started on tamoxifen. I remembered all the awful stories I'd heard over the past few months about its side effects, from both friends and strangers. But one step at time. Chemo was done. I tried to appreciate the real significance of this day. I had one more surgery to go, but the worst part was over.

Andrew helped me into the car and we headed home along the FDR. It was 6:00 P.M., and the sun was still shining, only just beginning to dip behind the skyscrapers of lower Manhattan. The days were getting longer and my mood was lifting. The thought *I am actually done* was still settling over me, and I let myself enjoy a true feeling of accomplishment as I looked at the intricate beauty of the Manhattan and Brooklyn bridges. Then another thought occurred to me: *I'm not just done. I've made it to the other side.* I was starting to feel a sense of hope and anticipation. Andrew was, too.

"You did it, baby, you're done," he said, looking over at me with a big smile and grabbing my hand. Even now, when I'm on the FDR driving my kids home from school, I see that view of the bridges and the East River and I remember. I remember how lucky I am to be alive, how strong I am, how much I've overcome, how much I've grown. It's my daily cue.

We pulled into our garage, but I was so weak that Andrew had to hold me, his arm linked through mine, as we walked into our building and rode silently up in the elevator. When it opened on our floor and I turned the corner, a wave of love and gratitude washed over me. Our door was completely covered with children's drawings and beautiful words of inspiration and love. "No More Chemo!" "You Make Me Strong." "You Are Brave." "We Are Proud of You." "The Woman You Are Makes Me Proud."

That last one made me laugh out loud. My little girls were so sweet, but how did they come up with these slogans?

The answer became obvious when we stepped inside. My mom and dad were right there, and I could picture them sitting around the table with my daughters, helping them create this heartwarming gift. And, of course, there were the final seventeen roses from Andrew, in a beautiful shade of coral. He also had a small box waiting for me. "Congratulations, baby," he said, handing it over. It was a watch I had been looking at when we took our Christmas trip to Turks and Caicos after my first round of chemo. Andrew had bought it when I wasn't looking and saved it all these months to give to me on this very special day.

EVEN THOUGH I felt horrible physically, I knew I had to go to work the next day. I was filling in for Robin, co-hosting *GMA,* and that responsibility was a great motivator when all I really wanted to do was curl up in a ball and stay in bed. But I had to keep on moving, which had been my mantra for the past six months. As Dr. Oratz had told me, "When you feel like taking a nap, go for a run, or at least a walk, instead."

I was in an exhausted fog of chemicals, but the adrenaline must have revived me. I was so excited to publicly mark the end of my breast cancer treatment. With my co-workers gathered around the desk, we showed the story looking back at my journey: from the mammogram all the way to the message I had taped the day before from my chemo chair. We showed a montage of every photo I had taken during treatment, rounds one through eight. *GMA*'s amazing social team had put together the beautiful collage with the hashtag "#BeBrave" in the lower right corner. Natasha struck the perfect tone, with my anthem,

"Brave" by Sara Bareilles, softly playing in the background, and ending with Andrew's video of Beth blowing her bubbles.

When we came back live, my colleagues had a surprise for me: They and the entire audience in Times Square had their own bottles of bubbles. I heard "Congratulations, Amy!" and watched the iridescent cloud rise over the studio.

"This is so beautiful," I said. "Thank you. And you know, while everyone's blowing these bubbles, I want to share something, because I had so much positive reaction on social media. . . ." We had put the chemo montage up on Facebook the day before, and comments had been pouring in. Women all across the country began tweeting me their chemo, radiation, and Herceptin photos with their fingers held up, counting off the rounds. We were united, in it together, and it was incredible.

"One of the responses stood out to me," I said. "Joanne Tamborough said, 'Congratulations. I, too, am a breast cancer survivor. Tough times don't last; tough people do.'"

"You are tough," said George Stephanopoulos.

"It just felt so inspiring to hear everyone else's stories. We're all in it together," I said.

As soon as I got home, I literally collapsed on my bed and slept for the rest of the day. Beth was right—I was in no condition to do any sort of celebrating. I stayed there for most of the weekend, trying to build up enough strength to go back to work on Monday.

Two weeks later, when May 8 came around, I was still weak but in a much better place to follow Beth's prescription. Kaitlyn had photographed the handwritten message and used it as an Evite to the celebration. The same friends who had gathered in early December to send me off into the uncharted waters of chemotherapy with "Amy's Last Hangover" returned to the Atlantic Grill to celebrate my making it to shore. Kaitlyn printed out lots of other pictures from the past twenty weeks; she even had cupcakes made with the pictures from each round of chemo printed in the frosting.

When I walked into the restaurant, I saw all the girls wearing T-shirts that said TEAM AMY on the front and, on the back, KICKING CANCER'S A**. My daughters still like wearing those cheeky shirts.

We were the same group, in the same corner of the same restaurant as last fall, but everything was different. Certainly I was different. I had not recovered physically from chemo—not even close—so I wasn't in the mood to drink much, but I was so happy to be there with some of my favorite people in the world.

That's the night I noticed how much my mom had changed, and not for the better. She looked thin, tired, and weak. She also looked scared. My mom had been remarkably strong from the initial diagnosis all the way through chemo, helping me keep my home together and taking care of my family—even the dog. She'd been with me almost every day for the past six months, basically moving in with us and going home only to switch out clothes and come back. But the weight of everything we'd been through had finally caught up with her. And the moment when the clear parameters of treatment were over, fear had set in. It was something I would wake up to myself a little later, but my mom felt it right away. I remember being mad at her that night—mad that she seemed so afraid, when all I wanted to do was relax and celebrate.

It was well into May before I felt my strength coming back, and it was the end of the summer when I began to see little sprouts of hair popping up all over my head. I'd lost about a third of my hair, and it was starting to grow back. The new strands looked like baby bird feathers and took about six months to catch up with the rest of my pixie cut. My eyebrows were filling back in, and my eyelashes were getting longer. I began to relax and loosen that tight white-knuckle grip I had placed over my thoughts and feelings, a constant squeeze to shut out any hopeful thoughts. Up until then I was too afraid to let myself imagine a day where I wouldn't be worried or fearful. But just then, I started to believe that the worst might be over, that I had a future, and it was bright.

Chapter Eleven

No Longer the Girl with the Ponytail

May always kicks off with one of my favorite annual events, the White House Correspondents' Dinner, that Washington tradition in which the press corps and members of government roast one another. I'd gone for the previous thirteen years, but this time it was like a graduation ceremony or a coming-out party, because I was done with chemo and determined to feel better and get back to being me, full-time. The problem was, I was still sick—really sick. The chemicals were still coursing through my bloodstream. At lunch the day of the dinner, I got so nauseated I had to run to the restaurant bathroom, leaving Andrew at the table. That night there were so many parties, but I didn't last long. We called it an early night. I felt depleted.

Andrew and I got up the next morning and went on my first post-chemo run, around the monuments and Tidal Basin. It was a beautiful day and I made it a full two miles, but I felt like I'd run a marathon. I remember wiping away tears out of frustration that I was still so weak.

May was going to be my month for resting, but it was also a turning point for me. Now that I was done with the part I'd dreaded most, I was ready to focus on giving back. This began with speaking publicly about my cancer battle.

On May 5, I received the Spirit of Life Award from City of Hope, a leading research and treatment center for cancer, diabetes, and other life-threatening diseases. My parents flew back to be with me for the big event at the Plaza. I took the girls out of school early, and we all sat at a big table with Andrew and many of my friends and colleagues who had helped me over the previous few months: Sara Haines; Melissa Lonner (my dear friend from NBC with the home in Turks and Caicos); Barbara Fedida; my assistant, Marly Faherty; Monica Coluso (who had organized hot meals for my family all throughout my chemo); and Kaitlyn Folmer. It was beautiful to look around the table and see all of them there for me once again. After lunch was the award presentation. Andrew introduced me. He was so brave, standing up in front of hundreds of people, wiping away tears as he described my fight over the last six months. He told the crowd that I was more than a cancer patient, that I was one of the happiest people he'd ever met, someone who loved life, her daughters and family, and peanut M&M's. He said I was strong and brave and that it was an honor to be my husband.

We were just coming out of the darkness, and his emotions were so raw, as were mine. My mom and I wiped away tears as we listened. When I walked to him to accept the award, the entire ballroom stood up, clapping. Andrew and I hugged and kissed, then I looked out at the audience in awe, taking it all in. I was proud. Proud of my husband, of my friends and family, and of *myself*. My lips were shaking with emotion as I smiled and said, "Thank you, thank you so much." I looked at my notes, summoned my courage, and began to share my story with the room. "One year ago, I could never have imagined I'd be standing here today, a cancer survivor. . . ."

Three days later I spoke at the United Nations, at a Moms +Social-Good conference sponsored by the Global Moms Challenge, an organization that works to improve the health and well-being of women and children. I shared the podium with Olivia Wilde, Elizabeth Smart, UN ambassador Samantha Power, Princess Zeid of Jordan, and Girl Scouts CEO Anna Maria Chávez, discussing education, the challenges and solutions involved with childbirth around the world, and how to inspire the next generation of global thinkers and leaders.

On May 14 I spoke at an event for Gilda's Club, a community organization for people living with cancer, and I'm proud to say that we raised over $350,000.

But I also worked that following weekend, doing an interview for *20/20* with Molly Bloom, the Poker Princess, in L.A. She was publishing a tell-all about her life running a celebrity poker game in Hollywood; she later moved the game to Wall Street, which brought her to the attention of the Russian mafia and, ultimately, the FBI.

It was a great interview, but when I got back, my mother sat me down and said, "What are you doing, Amy?"

She was worried that I was burning myself out. May was supposed to be my month to rest and recover, but I didn't seem to be slowing down, and my mom was upset. Okay, maybe the Poker Princess was not of earth-shattering importance, but I was actually turning down 50 percent of what I was being asked to do. And one of the reasons I love my job is that I occasionally get to cover the salacious, along with the stories that really matter. If I did only one or the other, I'd get bored. And if you're going to do it, you have to show just as much enthusiasm for celebrity headlines as you do for international affairs. You can't condescend. Besides, Molly Bloom marked my return to *20/20*. I'd cut back on pretty much everything except *Good Morning America,* and now I wanted to get back into the other shows, as well.

My speaking schedule was still pretty packed. On June 3, I spoke at the Susan G. Komen Impact Awards luncheon in the grand ballroom of the New York Hilton, where I was being honored for increasing cancer awareness.

But on June 9, after my body had had a few weeks to recover from chemo, I headed back to the hospital for reconstructive surgery. It would be natural to dread going back into the OR, but I couldn't wait to get those expanders out of me. I remembered feeling a similar way around week forty of my pregnancies: It doesn't even matter how bad the labor is; you just want that baby *out*.

Three times over the seven months the expanders were in, Dr. Choi had injected them with a huge syringe filled with saline, to pump them up and expand my skin and prepare it for implants. I went from basically nothing when I woke up from my mastectomy to a small A to a large A to a B, which is where I would stay.

When Andrew and I walked into NYU early that Monday morning, I was excited to be rounding this final lap, the last big thing on the list of tough physical procedures. The very same nurse who prepped me for surgery back in November was waiting for me once again. She gave me a big smile and said, "This is the fun one—you get new breasts! This is the good surgery." With that in mind, I smiled and drifted off without much fear or worry.

When I woke up, there was some pain, but nothing like the last time. Once again I had drains and stitches, outside and in. That's how they have to do it because the skin, after all it's been through, is very fragile. I spent that week in our house upstate. The kids were in school, but Andrew brought them back and forth from the city, and the middle of the woods was the perfect place for me to recuperate. You can't hear or see another human being from our home—only the occasional deer or turkey. The solitude took me far away from the doctors and the city and helped me to just *be* rather than *do*. There were a couple of long days where I felt a bit lonely, but it was important for me to let some of that depression in and simply experience it. As you may have noticed, I tend to overschedule, which is my coping mechanism; I stay busy to turn off my mind. But this week I left myself alone to watch movies, write in my journal, and read.

My body had changed, and looking in the mirror was, and still is, a constant reminder of all I've been through. I have a large visible scar under each breast, and there's an indentation in my right breast where Dr. Axelrod removed the bigger tumor. Dr. Choi decided to use "gummy bear" implants for my reconstruction. They get their name from the fact that they are pliable yet bounce back from touch. They have more structure than saline—the manufacturer touts that they're "form-stable"—and that's helpful when there's almost no natural tissue left from the mastectomy. Even as I write this, months later, I'm still wearing my grandma-like mastectomy bras. Underwire hurts my scars. But you know what? At that point, I wasn't worried about how anything looked. I was just so happy to feel like I was getting back to normal.

THERE WAS ONE aspect of my "new normal," though, that I was not expecting: to become engaged in a roiling controversy over the best approach to how we discuss and treat breast cancer.

In late June I took part in a Pfizer-sponsored event called "Beyond Pink." Five of us talked on a panel about our experience with the disease. It was my first encounter with a metastatic breast cancer patient, who had a very different perspective from mine and came out with guns blazing. You see, no one dies from breast cancer that remains in the breast. You die after metastasis, when the cancer spreads to different parts of the body, usually the bones, liver, lungs, and/or brain. Metastatic breast cancer patients are terminal.

"If one more person says, 'A mammogram saved my life,' I'm going to scream," she said. She was three panelists down from me on the dais. She knew my story. She knew who I was, and I thought, *Uh-oh*.

This woman had lived with cancer for ten years, but it had spread to her liver. She had already survived beyond the life expectancy for her condition, so I could only imagine her bitterness and frustration.

"I did everything right," she said. "Just like Ms. Robach. I caught my breast cancer early, or so I thought. I was young and the doctors told me they'd gotten it and everything was great and how lucky I was. Then ten years later it came back."

The discussion was very emotionally charged, which was understandable. What was harder to accept was the way I became a target for speaking out about the benefits of early detection. As the panel went on, I started to feel defensive. I didn't like the recurring implication that I was some kind of privileged snob who didn't know what cancer was really like. I listened to the harsh words and tried to let them pass me by.

But when it was time to wrap up, I reminded the audience that I was not naïve about what might lie ahead and that I did indeed know what it was like to have cancer. My parting line was, "I'm actually off to see my oncologist now. Today I begin the next phase of my cancer treatment: ten years of tamoxifen."

Over the new few weeks I would become increasingly aware of this very vocal community of metastatic patients who say that if it's going to come back, it's going to come back. In their view, it doesn't matter if the doctors intervened at stage 1 or stage 0 or stage 3. There's no way to know, they say, so to focus on early detection is putting money in the wrong place. They do not support Breast Cancer Awareness Month or the pink ribbon. They rally against increasing awareness and early detection. Most argue that instead of spending money telling women to get mammograms, those resources should be applied to the search for a cure and a way to stop cancer from spreading. They disagree with all the focus on early-stage breast cancer.

Immediately after the *People* article about me came out, Dr. Susan Love, a well-known surgeon who is very outspoken on issues of breast cancer, started blasting me on Twitter. I was still recovering from surgery, and she was appearing on my feed every five minutes.

By day two I called Kaitlyn and said, "Can you please block this woman from my Twitter account?" Our technical support team made sure I didn't have to see her nasty words again.

I'm in the public eye, and people are always taking potshots. Disagreeing with me is one thing, but I don't like it when they try to silence me, especially when they're being aggressively hostile. And it was even more disheartening when my only goal had been to spread hope, save lives, and raise money and awareness.

By this time I'd already gone to my boss, asking to do a series of reports on "girl power," about young women around the world who were speaking their minds and doing good, no matter who tried to stop them. The idea was to do maybe five or six profiles a year, on everyone from celebrities to unsung heroes, young women fighting battles here at home and around the world.

Heading my list: Malala Yousafzai, the teenager from the Swat Valley of Pakistan who'd become an advocate for girls' education, only to be shot in the head by the Taliban on her way to school. Malala miraculously recovered and spoke even *louder*. We learned she was planning a trip to Nigeria to bring attention to the plight of the more than two hundred girls who had been kidnapped by the Islamist group Boko Haram. Our bookers on *GMA* were already working with Malala's people to try to arrange coverage of her trip, as were the bookers for the *Today* show, and it was a heated competition. We had a series of meetings with representatives from the Malala Fund, and a few days later I got the email I'd been hoping for: "Congratulations. Mr. Lauer will be disappointed, but we're going to go with you and ABC News."

I was over the moon, but then I found out Malala was going to Nigeria on her seventeenth birthday, which was July 12—the week of my long-awaited girls-only trip to Italy.

I'd come up with the idea of a vacation right after round four of chemo, which had been the toughest of all. I'd just come back from Sochi, exhausted, and then we moved. I was surrounded by unpacked boxes as far as the eye could see, and I felt overwhelmed and hopeless, with nothing to look forward to except more needles and nausea and fatigue. Apparently my despair was contagious, because my daughters and my mom were soon mirroring it back to me.

One evening all of us were lying on the couch with the television flickering and no one really watching. I knew we needed something to lift us all out of this funk, and a thought popped in my head.

"What if," I blurted out, "when this is all over and behind me, we go somewhere, just girls, that we've never been to before, somewhere exotic."

My daughters screamed, "Yes!" and then, "Where?"

We brainstormed Hawaii, the Caribbean, and then . . . Italy. It sounds corny, but my daughters and I—as well as my girlfriends and I—have spent many nights watching and rewatching *Under the Tuscan Sun*. I've often joked that it's my dream to renovate an old estate in that part of the world and live happily ever after with vineyards and sunflowers all around me. That movie resonates with me because it's about overcoming something terrible (in the case of Diane Lane's character, a cheating husband and a divorce) and making something magical. It's about friendship and love and finding the perfect place to appreciate what really matters. I had so many girlfriends to thank for their incredible support, and this was going to be my way of giving back.

I'd started planning the next day. I would need close to a month to recover after my surgery before I could travel abroad. So, with the help of a travel agent, I picked a date and a villa and started creating the perfect vacation, which would commence right after *GMA* on Friday, July 4. I would be celebrating true independence that day, the freedom to reclaim my life after the absolute worst eight months I'd ever experienced.

Then, just a few weeks before the big day, I got the news about Malala. I had to make a tough choice to end my vacation three days early, reschedule five airline tickets, and eat the money I'd paid for those last nights at the villa. I spent a couple of days going over the pros and cons, but I couldn't help myself. I opted for the interview. My mom agreed to fly with my daughters back to New York; the other girls would go on to Rome for an extra two days; and Kaitlyn and I would fly to London and then on to Abuja, Nigeria.

Not only would I be interviewing Malala, I would also get to sit down with several of the girls who'd escaped Boko Haram's clutches and meet the parents of the girls still missing. It was an incredible story, and one that needed telling. I didn't want to spoil the vacation, but this was exactly the kind of story I'd gone into journalism to cover, a story that would have an impact and make people care.

I had another meeting with Dr. Oratz on June 26, and she cautioned me to take it easy. "Surgically you've been through a lot," she said. "You have to be careful. And remember, you can't lift anything for at least eight weeks."

But nothing could tamp down my mood when the time came to pack for this dual-purpose trip (although I let Andrew do the heavy lifting). My suitcase was a strange mix of sundresses and bathing suits for Tuscany and long pants and jackets for the mostly Muslim Nigeria.

My daughters, Kaitlyn, Sara Haines, and my NBC friends Jennifer Long, Melissa Lonner, and Kristine Johnson (now of CBS News) all flew together from New York, and my mom and Aunt Ann flew from Atlanta. We would meet up in Rome. As soon as I boarded that plane, I was *happy*. I felt my serotonin levels surge. I had my two daughters on either side of me—they made me sit in the middle—and my friends scattered throughout the plane. We watched movies, slept, and, before we knew it, we were in Rome. We had to wait only an hour to meet up with my mom and Ann, and the ten of us were off on our adventure.

The travel agent had scheduled several stops up the Mediterranean coast on our way to the villa, and the views were simply majestic—the cobalt-blue sea, the fig and olive trees, the summer sun. We stopped for a lunch of Italian wine, fresh warm bread with local olive oil, and homemade pasta. It was *exactly* as I hoped it would be.

And the villa was spectacular, just five kilometers outside the picturesque town of Siena. It overlooked its own vineyards and had a beautiful swimming pool. It even came with a house pet, Luca, a golden retriever, whom my daughters immediately blanketed with hugs.

We spent the next week touring small Tuscan towns, castles, vineyards, and shopping outlets. We even crashed a wedding at the neighboring villa. We only lasted ten minutes on the dance floor before we were found out and asked to leave. Yes, it was slightly embarrassing, but totally worth it. We've gotten a lot of mileage reliving that moment of reckless abandon. We ate most meals al fresco at a big table with more food than we could possibly handle, and each night we drank the villa's wine and talked and laughed until we were too tired to stay up a second longer.

Midway through the vacation, on a lazy, warm afternoon, I decided I would go on my first run since my reconstructive surgery. Dr. Choi had asked that I wait at least three weeks, and I had been patient and followed her orders. At last I felt like I was healed enough to go for it. And what better place to resume running than through the vineyards of Italy!

I've been an avid runner since high school. It's my outlet for almost everything. I run when I want to get out my frustrations, when I want to feel my strength, when I want to cry it out, or when I just want to be alone. I love the feeling of the wind on my face and music playing in my ears, my heart pounding, my legs racing. It's exhilarating. But this particular run was a special one. It was the first time since all the chemo chemicals had cleared my system. It was the first time since my final surgery. I was running on a new path, a path that had a real future.

As I turned and began making my way back to the villa, I thought I felt a thumping on the back of my neck—my ponytail. Instinctively, I reached back to grab it, but of course it wasn't there. Instead, my fingers brushed over my close-cropped boyish hair. I stopped running, put my hands to my knees, and tried to catch my breath. I was completely caught off guard. For one moment, I actually forgot all that I had been through this year. For one moment, I was my old self, on another run, like most days before I got cancer. Emotion flooded me, but as I fought back tears, I felt empowered. *Look at what you've accomplished in the past year,* I told myself. I was no longer the girl with the ponytail. In fact, I would never be the girl I was just a year ago. I would also never be the beaten-down, hopeless cancer patient I'd often felt like over the last eight months. I was a survivor. In that instant, I had hope and a vision of what I could still become. I realized I still had *time* to grow, *time* to make mistakes, and *time* to grow some more. Since the shock of my initial diagnosis, I hadn't let myself imagine the future, much less get excited about it. Time itself had become a frightening concept, but I told myself I would not let it frighten me anymore.

On our final night in Italy, I had a DJ come to the villa, and the ten of us danced until 2:00 A.M. We weren't under the Tuscan sun, but we were under a Tuscan supermoon, and it was perfect.

The next morning, my daughters, my mom and aunt, and two girlfriends piled into one car, headed to the Rome airport. My other friends and I drove into the city proper. Kaitlyn and I had a later flight to London and then the overnight flight into Abuja. But we still had some time to kill, so we spent a few fun hours sightseeing in Rome and, of course, ate one last incredible Italian meal before setting off for Nigeria.

Chapter Twelve

"To Avoid Criticism, Say Nothing"

The director of operations and communications at the Malala Fund, Eason Jordan, was waiting for us at Nnamdi Azikiwe International Airport. It was 5:00 A.M. in Nigeria, pitch black outside and overcrowded inside. Eason is a physically imposing man, strong and tall, with a security and journalism background. He co-founded Praedict, a war zone–focused security company, after ten of his CNN colleagues were killed in Iraq and Somalia. Eason wanted to empower people working in war zones to make lifesaving judgments about their movements and actions. We had met in New York over lunch a few weeks prior, to discuss security and logistics. That's when Eason insisted that he pick us up, a precaution I was thankful for when we arrived. We were bleary-eyed, but we quickly realized that we were not in Tuscany anymore.

Everywhere we looked, we saw soldiers with AK-47s. And although Abuja was considered the safest city in Nigeria, it was still Nigeria. There had been a bombing shortly before we arrived, which killed more than twenty people who'd been watching a World Cup game on television, and the World Cup finals were still going on. Eason was at heart a Southern gentleman—he hailed from Georgia—and he escorted us quickly to our waiting vehicle.

As we emerged from the terminal into the thick, heavy air, the smell of wood smoke filled my lungs. We climbed into an SUV and sped down the highway toward our hotel, and I was struck by the number of people walking along the highway, miles from any discernible destination. There were hardly any other cars on the four-lane highway, just dozens and dozens of men and women walking along the shoulder.

When we finally turned in through the hotel gates, the sun was beginning to rise, and we were greeted by guards with machine guns and bandoliers wrapped across their chests. One of them made our driver pop open the rear hatch. They inspected our entire vehicle, even the undercarriage and the trunk, and eventually let us inside the protected compound. From there we all went to our rooms and slept for a few hours, awaiting Malala's arrival.

Before we left for Italy and Nigeria, Kaitlyn and I had met with Jon Williams, the head of international coverage at ABC, and he told us the rule of thumb in Abuja: "If you leave the hotel, never stay in one place more than ten minutes." The fact was, Boko Haram was everywhere, and American broadcasters made excellent targets. So we'd said no publicity beforehand. We didn't want anyone to know that Malala was going to be in the country. We didn't even want anyone to know that I was going to be in the country.

Our plan was to interview the girls who had escaped from their kidnappers, and then we'd speak with Malala. Afterward, we were going to meet with the families of the girls who were still being held. Obviously we knew there were risks, so we had to work out the logistics very carefully. We needed our own security detail, but Nigeria doesn't allow anyone to carry weapons except members of the military, and the military had been infiltrated by Boko Haram. So while the Malala Fund was paying these guys to protect us, Boko Haram could be paying them to shoot up the place and bring us back as hostages. We were placing a lot of trust in these soldiers, and I hoped we'd picked the right ones.

We were ready to roll with lights, cameras, and microphones when Malala's entourage arrived. The group included her father, Ziauddin, a school principal and himself a seasoned campaigner for education, and Shiza Shahid, the young and beautiful Stanford grad and McKinsey consultant who'd become Malala's chief strategist while she was in the hospital recovering from the gunshot wound to her head.

Wrapped in bright and beautiful scarves, wearing traditional Pakistani clothing, Malala walked into the front lobby and gave a sheepish smile to the waiting press.

"Happy birthday," I said.

"Thank you," she replied.

My team and I arranged to have a quick one-on-one with her before she headed out for a birthday dinner in the hotel, leading up to our big sit-down the following day with the kidnapped girls' families and several girls who had escaped. Malala was gracious and humble, but she also had the feisty force of a teenager. I loved her from the moment I met her and couldn't help but think how incredible it was to be meeting someone who would most likely follow in the footsteps of her beloved role model, Benazir Bhutto, to become the prime minister of Pakistan. The moment Malala started speaking, I could sense that she was motivated by the responsibility to lead, and it was evident that this teenager is up for all the challenges and difficulties that a calling entails. She is wise beyond her years, and yet there were brief moments when I saw the teenager in her. That mischievous look in her eyes gave her away. She was, after all, only seventeen.

"I can't wait until I turn eighteen," she told me, "when I will be able to travel alone. I should like to get a one-seater car, so I can go places on my own, with no one watching over me." For now her father, understandably, doesn't let her out of his sight. But full independence is what she is fighting for, for all the women around the world and especially for the women in her own country.

Malala spoke with me about the need for educating all girls. "If countries would like to be powerful, they should stop buying weapons and invest in education," she said. She smiled as best she could, her face partially paralyzed by a Taliban bullet. In that now-signature half smile, you see a young girl who has faced fear, beat the odds, and stood back up in direct defiance of the terrorists who wanted her dead—who still want her dead. She said, "The Taliban tried to silence one girl's voice, and instead they heard the voices of hundreds of thousands." The power of her words still rocks me when I reread them.

Malala has faced an extreme example of what so many of us encounter (in much smaller ways) each and every day. How easy it is for our critics to silence us, change us, define us. Here is an inspiration with a lesson for us all: Never be quieted by the haters. The next few days were filled with incredible voices of courage and resilience, and I left with a new appreciation for the power of the human spirit.

I FLEW HOME on July 15, and went to work the next day with a fever of 101. This was only a couple of weeks before the Ebola outbreak in West Africa really hit the news. If my timing had been a little different, I would have been hustled off to an isolation unit at the CDC in Atlanta or to a special containment unit in Omaha.

But just being sick was bad enough. I had cramping that was worse than giving birth, and felt like I was going to throw up at any moment. As usual, I called my brother, but he didn't answer, and neither did my doctor. So I called my dad.

He told me, "Actually, I'm at the CDC right now. Hang on . . ." Then he came back on the line and asked me about my symptoms, where I'd been, and when I'd eaten last. His diagnosis: "Salmonella. I'm pretty sure of it. You need to get on Cipro right away."

I'd been out of the studio for weeks, so I felt like I really needed to get back to work, but the fever didn't break for three days. With the help of antibiotics, I tried to sleep it off, but I also had a dental appointment for the girls and myself, which I'd had to schedule six weeks in advance. I pulled myself out of bed, herded the girls onto the subway, and went up to our old neighborhood to see Dr. Lee Gold.

I waited in my semiconscious state while the girls went first. They got their cleanings, X-rays, and sealants put on their teeth. It seemed to take forever, as I slumped down farther in the chair, feeling ever more feverish.

When it was finally my turn to go in, I figured it would be short and sweet, despite the fact that I'd bailed on my last appointment because of all I'd been going through with breast cancer. The hygienist did my cleaning, and then Dr. Gold came in to give me the all clear, but he kept looking at the roof of my mouth. He began to mutter about something on my palate.

I was so sick it took me a second to realize where he was headed with this. But then he got my attention. He held up a mirror, asked me to open wide, and pointed out the small mass.

Dr. Gold knew I'd just wrapped up chemotherapy, so he had a hard time looking me in the eye as he said, "Hate to tell you this, but you're going to have to have this checked out."

I groaned. "Not again."

"You're not a smoker, right?"

"I'm not a smoker."

"It's probably nothing, but you'll need to see a maxillofacial surgeon to have it removed. And then a biopsy."

I was so tired, it was all I could do not to decompensate right there in the dental chair. I was reeling but doing my best to stay calm. I didn't want Dr. Gold to see how terrified I was, how *angry* I was that I had to face this now, so soon after everything else. He gave me the surgeon's card, and I called immediately to set up an appointment for the next day.

The worst part was that Andrew was traveling again, so it was very déjà vu—me being alone, and another doctor telling me I needed a biopsy. The only thing that kept me going was the fact that my daughters were with me. But even so, physically weak and now mentally entertaining every possible worst-case scenario, I didn't make it far—to the middle of Broadway between Houston and Prince, one of the craziest and most annoying streets in all of New York—before I broke down completely, sobbing on the sidewalk as throngs of people surged around us.

But my girls were amazing. They rubbed my back and asked what was wrong. I didn't want to scare them, but I went with the truth.

"It's probably not a big deal," I said. "Mommy's just feeling really tired. And they found a little bump on the roof of my mouth that needs looking into."

"You're going to be okay, Mom," Ava told me. "No one would let this happen twice. It's not going to be cancer, so don't worry."

I felt so weak and so small for burdening them with this, but Andrew wasn't around, so it fell to my eleven-year-old to do the comforting.

As soon as I got home, I did a Google search for "tumor, roof of mouth." The first thing that came up: palate cancer. Very successful if treated early, unless it's spread to the lungs. I burst into tears—again.

Getting over salmonella was now the least of my worries. I was pissed that I had to go through this all over again, all the worry and fear. Enough already!

I saw a specialist on Monday, July 18, and had the excision and biopsy on July 21. If you've ever chomped down on a brittle cracker caught sideways in your mouth, then you can imagine how much it hurts to have an incision on the roof of your mouth. And then they had to cauterize—burn—it, because they couldn't put stitches there.

"You won't be able to go to work probably for a couple days," the surgeon said. "It'll hurt to talk."

"You've got to be kidding me," I said. But he was right about the pain. "As soon as you get the results, will you please call me?"

"Absolutely, absolutely."

I subsisted on lukewarm soup and yogurt, and I had to rinse with a numbing solution for two weeks, but I didn't miss a day of work. As always, I needed to stay busy while I kept checking in with the nurse.

"Nope. We don't have it yet."

I went in a week later for the results, and my heart was beating like a jackhammer. "Good news," the doctor said. "The growth was benign."

This time I didn't cry, but tears welled in my eyes, and I said to myself, "Thank God." I was still busy fighting my last battle.

ON JULY 26, writer Peggy Orenstein wrote an op-ed in *The New York Times* arguing against contralateral prophylactic mastectomy, the very surgery I'd had. She referred to me by name and used the quote I'd given to *People,* where I said I'd taken the more aggressive approach of having both breasts removed because I wanted to stay alive for my kids, that I wanted to "be at my daughters' graduations. I want to be at their weddings. I want to hold my grandchildren." Orenstein put forth statistics showing that, in most cases, removing "the other breast" just to be safe had no effect on survival. She made no mention of the fact that, in my case, it had been *exactly* the right thing to do— that, in fact, my breast had harbored pre-cancerous cells, and thus my situation was actually the living counterargument to her point. I reached out through ABC's vice president of communications, Heather Riley, saying that we wished she had contacted me before quoting me and using my story. She fired back with a flaming email to Heather that really knocked me back on my heels.

"It may well be that Ms. Robach would survive her disease even if she had bumped into her tumor in the shower when it became clinically apparent. It may also be (and again I apologize for my directness) that her cancer, despite treatment, will return," she wrote. "She simply doesn't know at this point and continually saying that the mammogram saved her life is simplistic and disrespectful to many women living with cancer." She asked that I stop saying that cancer made me a "better" person, because, she said, I was hurting the people who need my advocacy the most. I was fuming. Who was she to tell me what to *feel*? This was my story, my cancer, my life.

It took three weeks for the pain to subside from the roof of my mouth, and even now there's a sensitive hole where the benign mass once grew. All the while, I had been easing into my tamoxifen regimen, slowly increasing the dose, and by August 7 I was up to the full twenty milligrams a day. That's when the side effects really kicked into high gear. It was also the day I flew to Atlanta after *GMA* to try to line up a booking with Justin Ross Harris, the dad accused of leaving his toddler son to die in a hot car while he sexted teenage girls with photos of his genitals.

I was talking over dinner with Lawrence Zimmerman—the attorney for Justin's wife, Leanna—and Lawrence's wife, when I had my very first hot flashes. I felt a wave of intense heat wash over my entire body, my head, my face. My back began to sweat. Nice. I was hoping no one noticed. Sweat has a funny way of making people appear nervous or untrustworthy—never a prime quality in a journalist. I was neither of those things; I was just in hormonally induced menopause! Thankfully, *if* they noticed, they didn't say a word.

As usual, I was zigging and zagging between covering the important issues of the day and foraying into the sordid and sensational. And then, only a few days later, those categories converged in another attack on me that, despite the author's credentials, had all the earmarks of the worst form of tabloid journalism.

On August 12, *New York* magazine's website published a piece called "Avoiding the Breast Cancer 'Warrior' Trap." It was written by a physician from Sloan Kettering, Dr. Peter Bach, whom I remembered from the Gilda's Club meeting where I'd spoken in May. He'd actually introduced himself to me at the event. He told me his wife had died at an all-too-early age of breast cancer, and we spent several minutes together, one-on-one, as I expressed my sorrow and commiserated with him. What I didn't know was that he'd been taking copious notes during my speech. And apparently what I said really annoyed him. I've never been clear, though, why he chose to use me as a whipping boy.

For starters, he referred to my "recent brush" with breast cancer, as if I'd somehow gotten off easy. I don't know about you, but I would never refer to someone who had two malignant tumors and a positive node, who had undergone two major surgeries and six months of debilitating chemotherapy, as having had a "brush" with a disease. He then referred to my speaking about my experience as telling "a story about cancer that is both wrong and hurtful." I'm sorry, but how can my personal story, told truthfully, ever be wrong? After which he assumed the full mantle of authority by saying, "I should know. I'm a doctor at a cancer hospital."

Nothing wrong with that, but then, as if to highlight the difference between a highly credentialed expert like himself and a mere television personality, this is how he chose to describe me: "Every inch the network TV star with four-inch heels, runway model legs, a Mentos smile, and a light Southern lilt wrapping broadcaster's diction, Robach was off track right from the start. A mammogram saved her life, she told us. But that is not something she could possibly know."

Now, going on about a woman's looks in a serious discussion is usually a way of belittling her intelligence, but, beyond that, the American Cancer Society concurs with my position on early screening for women forty and up. Obviously, other corners of the cancer world hold other points of view, but Dr. Bach said my advocacy for early screening "trampled over this rich debate" and equated my description of my personal choice with "misinformation." As I've said, he may have disagreed with me based on large clinical samples, but in my case there can be no doubt that it was 100 percent the right thing to do.

He also said that my talking about fighting back against cancer implied that women who die "must be dying for their lack of fortitude." Where did he get that? He offered a strained analogy about boxing—fighters versus slackers—and medieval ideas of finding salvation through self-mutilation. Then, most hurtful of all, he asserted that by urging women to get screened early, I was blaming women who didn't get an early mammogram for their own disease. Nothing could be further from the truth. He twisted my words of optimism and encouragement to fit his own preconceived narrative.

I found the piece to be so over the top, and such a demeaning and personally hostile attack, that I was flabbergasted. It was as if because I look a certain way and am on television, I deserved none of the compassion (or even common courtesy) he purports to offer the millions of other women who have breast cancer. Also galling was the fact that he wrapped himself in the sacred banner of evidence-based medicine and hardheaded epidemiology but still played the sympathy card on his own behalf, at the same time ending with one more dig at me for the way I look. Yes, his own wife died of breast cancer, for which I had already expressed my deepest sympathies. But his tagline? "I know of what I speak. My wife also looked great in heels."

I'd been so happy about that speech and proud that we'd raised so much money, and now he was trying to take that away from me. But as I was discovering, there's a metastatic breast cancer community that is very angry and dislikes the fact that so much attention is focused on early detection. Many take offense at the message of bravery or the fighter imagery. They don't even like the term "survivor." *Who are you to call yourself a survivor?* they might say. *You don't know that you've survived.* Or, *My mom died. Does that mean she wasn't a fighter?*

People are hurting, and they want to lash out. But I have never advocated double mastectomy for anyone but me. It was my choice, and it ended up being a potentially lifesaving one, because that second tumor and pre-cancerous tissue hadn't shown up in my mammogram.

And as for mammograms, I think it's outrageously irresponsible for anyone to say that women should wait until they're fifty. Peter Bach said screening at forty would save only one in two hundred breast cancer patients—but that's ten thousand women! How is that an "only"? Not to mention that I was one of those women saved by early detection.

After twenty years in front of the camera, I'm used to mean tweets and criticism. They come in a daily barrage. But I have to admit that Dr. Bach's article hit me hard. I rummaged through my memory bank for some of the quotes that had sustained me during other attacks. I love this quote attributed to Winston Churchill: "You have enemies? Good. That means you've stood up for something, sometime in your life." And Aristotle: "To avoid criticism, say nothing, do nothing, be nothing."

I'm sure the speech I gave at Gilda's Club wasn't perfect. I was still in a chemo fog, and I came back to the imagery of being a "warrior" against the disease, and perhaps I was a little too *rah, rah, I'm going to get through this fight!* But I don't take back anything I said, because in that moment it all felt real and true, and because other people who'd been through it could relate. I wasn't getting paid for that speech; I was just trying to provide some succor and inspiration for the other women in the room. And for that, Peter Bach tried to paint me as an idiotic cheerleader. In no way was I saying that we shouldn't create more of a voice for people who've lost hope and that we shouldn't do more to fund research into all phases of the disease. But that doesn't take away from the importance of prevention and early detection.

By the way, I'm supremely aware of the fact that I could be joining the ranks of those with end-stage metastatic cancer. I'll know in the next five to fifteen years, and, believe me, I hear the clock ticking in my head. I don't know that it'll ever stop. The chance of cancer coming back right now is 16 percent, and it significantly decreases if I make it to fifty-two. That is a long time for me to keep on living. And, as Andrew says, even if the worst happens, there's no need to die before you die.

On August 18 I was given the honor of moderating a conference with UN Secretary-General Ban Ki-Moon and Malala on the importance of educating women worldwide. I brought my daughters, and it was thrilling to see them sitting in the front-row seats where the delegates usually sit. Truth be told, they weren't all that excited. But I told them, "When you look back at this ten years from now, you'll so be happy you were here."

I wanted my girls to meet this seventeen-year-old who'd stared down the Taliban. At the UN that day, her message was concentrated into what had become her rallying cry: "If a country wants to be powerful, then invest in education, not weapons."

A few months later, Malala would share the 2014 Nobel Peace Prize. She'd already accomplished so much, and yet the attempts to silence her kept on coming. Anytime I checked on Twitter, there was a die-hard group of commenters saying horrible things like, "What about Gaza?" and "You're a traitor!" But at that time it mostly just felt therapeutic for me to see this girl, less than half my age, face all that hostility and still be smiling, standing, talking, and spreading her message.

I went from the UN forum straight to Times Square, to do an interview that I thought was going to be a zigzag from Malala. Taylor Swift was debuting a new single, and I prepared myself for a major tonal shift from empowerment to teen angst. But I was surprised by what happened next. Once Taylor and I got going, I felt a thread of connection. Taylor and Malala were both young women with immense followings for completely different accomplishments, but both embodied girl power: They kept speaking (or singing) despite what others might think, say, or write.

The title of Taylor's song was "Shake It Off." It's a catchy dance tune, but if you listen to the lyrics, it's also a simple, potent message for anyone who's taken a few hits, whether from high school bullies or cancer—or cancer-patient advocates with a different point of view. "Shake It Off." For damn sure that's what I needed to do.

After the interview, I told Taylor, "I know why you wrote the song. But I hope you know how important and meaningful it is for *everyone* who listens to it." I added, "This was exactly what I needed to hear today. I've had the voice of a mean critic stuck in my head on repeat, but now I'm just going to sing your song to drown it all out."

Taylor seemed genuinely touched. She said, "Thank you for telling me that. It's exactly what I was hoping to accomplish."

Then again, shaking it off is never as easy as you think, so going forward I wanted to be fully informed. I had to make sure my message was medically correct and that I was doing the right thing by speaking about the benefits of early detection, so I consulted a few experts. I forwarded the *New York* post to my oncologist, Dr. Oratz, and to Dr. Larry Norton, the deputy physician-in-chief for breast cancer programs at Memorial Sloan Kettering. They told me that Dr. Bach's words were appalling and offensive, and they agreed with me that early detection does save lives.

Dr. Norton went so far as to share what he called "a few thoughts that have served me well in similar circumstances."

On "warrior": Not all fighters win, but all those who surrender are sure to lose.

On "celebrating survival": Celebrating victors does not equate to dishonoring the fallen.

On "continuing the battle": Those who do well (because of modern science and medicine, including screening) have an obligation to do everything they/we can to help others do well. Not everyone will, but that doesn't mean that we shouldn't try.

On "What is the most important way one can help others?": Everything—research, education, support, encouragement—is important. What is the most "important" part of the airplane? The fact that all the pieces of the airplane work together.

Andrew decided to pen a letter to the editor of the magazine that had put Dr. Bach's comments online. He wanted to defend me, and, in the end, writing it was cathartic for both of us, but we decided against sending it. We didn't want to extend a flame war, with opposing forces simply yelling at each other (and never listening), á la Jerry Springer. But I'll include it here, where I can provide context.

Many of the offensive tweets I've received over the last year come from women who have metastatic breast cancer. Many of these women are terminal, but as John Irving famously said, "We are all terminal cases." I know that one day I may be among the 30 percent of breast cancer patients who become metastatic, and I also know that it is in everyone's interest to band together to share resources and funding. We are so much stronger together than we ever could be divided into factions. We can promote prevention and early detection and at the same time raise money to fund the researchers around the world to find a cure for metastatic breast cancer. It's not a question of either/or. It's both/and—always.

So here's Andrew's letter:

To the editor: When you read an article by a doctor about breast cancer, you may have certain expectations—to come away with some additional knowledge of this dreaded disease, to have a greater understanding of what it's like to battle it, to learn about a new advance in treatment. At least that's what we hope to hear from our doctors, the very people who are, quite literally, lifesavers. What you do not expect to see is a personal attack on a victim of breast cancer who the doctor has never examined or met. The piece authored by Dr. Peter Bach on August 12 reads just like that—a personal attack on ABC news anchor Amy Robach. Robach has been fighting for her life while at the same time sacrificing her privacy to help inform others on the reality of breast cancer. The words and tone that Dr. Bach used were extremely inappropriate, hurtful, harmful, and, in the end, dishonorable.

Criticizing a woman, any woman, and the way she decides to handle this awful disease is not the way I would ever expect any medical professional to act. Especially not one who claims to be an expert on the subject and whose own family has been devastated by this disease. The fact that Dr. Bach would go on to use Robach's femininity and appearance as a tool to diminish her for the purpose of his argument leaves me speechless. He goes on to belittle Robach for saying "a mammogram saved my life," arguing she can't possibly know that. Well, he can't possibly know that it didn't.

Over the course of my treatment, I received incredible letters and emails—thank-you notes, really. Women wrote that my story had inspired (or scared) them into scheduling long-avoided mammograms. At least a dozen revealed that it was *that* mammogram that uncovered their cancer.

It was incredible to know that my personal tragedy could be empowering for others, but one card stood out. It was from Mount Pleasant, South Carolina, the coastal town just outside Charleston where I'd lived when I was a cub reporter at WCBD-TV 2 Action News. Deb Greig, mother of two and former news director of the ABC affiliate in Charleston—my competition when I was down there—wrote that she'd followed my career and made a point of watching *GMA* to see how I was doing. She also said that she'd been watching on November 11, 2013, when I announced that I had cancer. After hearing my story, she felt an immediate sense of urgency and ran out to her car to pull out a crumpled mammogram prescription she'd shoved in her glove box months earlier. That morning, she called her doctor on her way to work and scheduled her overdue mammogram for the next day. As it turned out, her diagnosis was similar to mine, and she thanked me for saving her life. She'd had a double mastectomy on Christmas Eve, and with her two daughters by her side, she was now recovering and cancer-free.

Because of our Charleston connection, I was especially touched by Deb's story, and I wanted to meet her and her two daughters. The perfect opportunity arose as *GMA* prepared for its annual Go Pink Day on October 1, 2014, the first anniversary of my own lifesaving mammogram. I hopped on a plane with Kaitlyn and my other producer, Rich McHugh, and we headed south.

As soon as we walked out of Charleston International Airport, the familiar warm, salty air blanketed me. I used to call it hot, humid pea soup, but on this day I was surprised at how good it felt to be back. We set up our interview at the Planters Inn, in one of the many spectacular garden courtyards Charleston is so famous for. Deb and I hugged as soon as we saw each other, and I met her two beautiful daughters. She took me through her own wrenching diagnosis, which had taken place just days after my own. Then she talked about the heartbreak I knew all too well: telling her two grown daughters she had breast cancer. But for Deb, it was even more difficult. Her ex-husband—her daughters' father—had died suddenly of lung cancer the year before.

"I didn't think life could be that cruel," she told me, "that my daughters would lose another parent to this awful disease."

That's why Deb told me she would be forever grateful that I had shared my experience on that day in November. Here I was, sitting across from three wonderful women, all of us changed by breast cancer. We were all wounded, no doubt, but we had grown so much stronger over these past few months. And we were smiling. That's what struck me—how happy we were to be there together, how happy we were to be alive.

Deb's story was set to air on October 1, but I also had something else very special to help usher in *GMA* Goes Pink Day. The morning before, on September 30, I'd headed straight off the set to fly down to Hartsfield-Jackson Atlanta International Airport. There, I went into the bathroom to change my clothes, then boarded another plane. But not just any plane. Delta Airlines had donated a jumbo jet with a pink belly to fly one hundred fifty cancer survivors—and my new best friends—up to New York. They christened it Breast Cancer One, and they'd been making this trip in support of Breast Cancer Awareness Month for ten years, joining forces with BCRF, Breast Cancer Research Foundation.

I walked on board in my custom pink Delta flight attendant uniform. "Good afternoon, ladies," my fellow flight attendant (the legit one) announced. "We have a special guest flight attendant on this afternoon's flight to New York City. Please welcome *Good Morning America*'s Amy Robach."

Each beautiful woman was on her feet, clapping and cheering, pink boa flying up in the air.

I got on the intercom and said, "Thank you so much. I am so excited to be on Breast Cancer One with all of you. I want to hear all of your stories and celebrate the fact that we're all here together today, but first I want to invite every one of you to Times Square tomorrow morning to join me on *GMA*. Who's up for it?"

You can imagine the response. I went down the aisle, kissing, hugging, sharing smiles, and snapping selfies. I served food and lots of bubbles, but mostly I listened to the stories of dozens and dozens of women. Some were on that plane against all odds, in the middle of their treatments. Some were bald, and some wore wigs or bandannas, but they were there, and they were all wearing smiles. Big ones. These women were not here to complain, to moan about their aches and pains, to lament the loss of their breasts, their hair, their femininity. Instead, they lifted one another up, supported one another, danced and sang, cheered and hollered, all while wearing crowns, high heels, and lipstick. These women refused to let cancer define them or take one more thing away from them. They were fighters—warriors, even—and the most impressive group of women I have ever met. I was humbled to be among their ranks.

This is not to say there weren't tears that day, but they weren't from sadness. Ever since I was little, my mom has always said, "Tears are powerful; never apologize for them." On that plane, I saw powerful, kick-ass tears, filled with determination and spunk.

Some women told me their "number," as in "I'm a two-year survivor" or "I'm a ten-year survivor." Which got me thinking. Where do I mark my one-year anniversary? Is it when I had my mastectomy? Or when I finished chemo?

One woman told me, "I started counting from the day I found out I had cancer, because that's the day I started surviving."

Bam. I had my answer.

The fact is, I'd already begun to feel quite a bit of anxiety about how I was going to get through October 30, the anniversary of the day the doctors told me I had breast cancer, which was fast approaching. It was weighing not only on me but on my mom. She'd been talking to her therapist, trying to figure out what she was going to do that day. And she'd started dreading the sound of the phone.

"If it rings that day," she said, "I'm going to lose it, because it'll just take me back to that moment when the phone rang and it was you telling me you had cancer."

So I began to wonder out loud: "What am I going to do on that day? Am I going to sit around and feel sorry for myself? Am I going to binge-watch chick flicks?"

Then Kaitlyn had a brilliant idea, as she so often does. Our dear friend Sara Haines was getting married, and I'd been thinking about throwing her a shower.

"Make the day about somebody else," Kaitlyn said. "How about Sara's shower?"

The idea was so perfect, it was like slipping into my favorite sweater—all warm and fuzzy. Take the anniversary of bad news and make it about new beginnings, about celebrating life and the years to come and all the wonderful things that marriage embodies.

I invited a couple of dozen women to my place and ordered food from the Irish restaurant down the street; there were cupcakes with Sara and her fiancé Max's picture on them. We covered the apartment with pink and white balloons that we lifted from a Taylor Swift event on *GMA* that morning (hey, I call it being green!).

My daughters love Sara like nobody's business, so they were there and especially thrilled to be up at 10:00 P.M. on a school night. Half of *GMA* came, too. "Hello," I said. "Who's putting on the show tomorrow?" We all wound up dancing in the kitchen to S Club 7 and Backstreet Boys, which I tend to think is a good marker of a party's success.

Later, Sara told me there was a moment when she saw this carefree look on my face, which she said was the same face I'd had in Tuscany—my "pre-cancer" expression. The fact is, I wasn't thinking about my diagnosis, or my odds for survival, or where I was a year ago and how much had changed. I was totally in the moment, and I was totally happy.

"I want to spend my life looking forward to the next chapter," I told her.

Epilogue

Beauty in Every Instant

For women who've been successfully treated for breast cancer, there is a 30 percent chance that the disease will come back. There's also something called an "Onco Score," which weighs the details of each case to arrive at an individual's specific odds of a recurrence. My Onco Score predicts my chances of bad news at 16 percent. But as my brother explained to me, the odds for any given individual are either 100 percent or zero percent. That's because, where it counts, each of us is a population of one.

The disease gets cut out and blasted and poisoned away, and then you sit and wait. Doctors say, "You're going to be fine," but it really breaks down into survival rates at five years and survival rates at ten years. If breast cancer metastasizes, it's terminal. I've always been a very positive person, even during my divorce and earlier medical issues. I'm like Orphan Annie, I guess, always believing that everything's going to be better tomorrow, even when it's hitting the fan today.

But when I was diagnosed, I felt that my sunny outlook had been stolen, and for a long time I was pissed that I couldn't get it back. I kept trying to frame things in a positive way, but somehow I couldn't find the unbridled joy and optimism I used to have. That's because, deep down, I spent a lot of my time feeling terrified.

Fear is an adaptation meant to keep us out of trouble, so it can be a good thing, but only if we learn how to manage it and make the most of what it's trying to tell us. But there have been plenty of moments since my diagnosis when what I felt was plain old vanilla fear, and that's when I'd break down.

Living with cancer is like your first time on a sailboat: If you're not used to sailing, it takes a while to adjust to the way the boat heels over on its side. It takes time to relax and accept that this is just how sailboats are and that you're not going to go down because you're on a slant and a few waves are coming over the railing.

When you're living with cancer, your feet can be on dry and solid ground, but you still feel tippy. You are never fully stable and secure. I've always been a list-maker, a goal-setter, and a forward thinker, because I've always had the luxury of assuming that the future is part of the deal. I felt robbed of that, as well. For the first time in my life, I was afraid to think about next year, or the year after. Trying to picture five or ten years down the road seemed impossibly audacious. I've had to work to see the future as part of the excitement of life, and that excitement comes not only from anticipating it but from investing in it, too.

I think we all begin to see mortality as less distant and abstract as we get older. Our expectations no longer flow endlessly from this decade to the next and on and on. Instead, we start counting backward, keeping a tally of how much time we figure we might have left. When I got my diagnosis, that sense of limited time hit me in the face with a whopping one-two punch.

So for a while I stopped making to-do lists and caring about whether the laundry was neatly folded. But indifference to the small stuff is unsettling when being super-organized and getting all those details right is essential to who you are.

Technically, a breast cancer patient is back to "normal" after a year out of chemo. But the fear lingers in your gut *because you're only good until you find that next lump, or that next ache, or you do the next blood work. You no longer have the luxury of feeling that tomorrow is a given.*

When *I am going to die* becomes front and center in your consciousness, you lose touch with the little pleasures of moment-to-moment existence. The cup of coffee in the morning isn't as tasty, and going to bed at night isn't as cozy, because you've looked beyond the veil. Once you've lost the positive illusion of endless time, you have to struggle to feel that life is good, because you can never say to yourself, *Relax. Settle in. I'm going to be here awhile.*

There have been a lot of days since October 2013 in which I've felt in my gut that my cancer will come back. But, as Andrew always reminds me, "Don't die before you die." Every day I try to bring my focus back to the beauty of life rather than the fear of death.

In books and movies, characters who have a health crisis always quit their high-powered jobs to do something "more meaningful," like work with wood or grow organic vegetables. But you don't have to completely reinvent yourself in a one-stoplight town in order to be transformed by a horrible experience. I would say that there's also something called "transformation in place." It's more subtle, because it looks like you're doing the same things. But the difference is, you're doing all those things in a more mindful way, because you've looked into the valley of death.

The issue isn't whether your life is hectic or low key but whether it is authentically *yours*. Whether I have five years or another fifty, I want to relish every minute. And for me, that means living in the moment and doing exactly what I do, and at the same frenetic pace, because I really love it. I think the way I've lived my life has helped me cope with cancer. I mean, I'm used to getting up and putting on a big smile on days when I feel like crap and just want to hide under the covers.

I've spent my whole life jumping onto planes and working crazy hours and getting no sleep, and even before I had cancer, I spent many nights in a hotel feeling completely torn up by the fact that I wasn't with my children. When I was diagnosed, my guilt was compounded by a "blame the victim" feeling, as if I had done something to deserve my disease. With all the talk about the health effects of stress and diet, I thought, *This is the hand of God. This is karma.*

But over time I've come back to this: I've always followed my heart. When I'm working, I'm happy, and I choose to believe—and I hope I'm right—that my daughters will look back and say, *My mom followed her passion. We were loved and always taken care of. But she never gave up what she loved for us.* I've made mistakes as a mom and as a woman, and I've questioned things like spending weeks away from my kids in the middle of chemo and putting my health at risk by going to Sochi. I don't want them to feel the kind of guilt I sometimes do. I hope my daughters will say with pride, *Look what my mom did.*

I'm raising my girls to be successful, independent, happy human beings. My job has forced the independence part, because I am definitely not helicoptering around, ready to swoop down at any minute to fight their battles for them. They know they're expected to work hard and to achieve to the best of their abilities. They know they have my support, but they also know they have to do it for themselves.

I've always played to win. When I got my first network job, the people I started out with in Charleston said to me, "You always told us you were going to make it to New York. Holy crap, you actually did it." But I did it in part by being so eager to please that I became a bit of a joke. Whenever somebody was asked to work all night or go out in a hurricane, they'd say, "Who do you think I am, Amy?"

Cancer has helped me get beyond being such a pleaser. I've learned to stand up for myself and to not be quite so invested in winning people over.

In a weird way, cancer set me free, because I can now say no to things that I would never have before. When I was in the middle of treatment, I realized for the first time that I could walk away from this job that I'd been working toward my whole life, and I could be happy.

My biggest professional triumph—landing the news anchor position at *GMA*—occurred during the one six-month period when I was not engrossed in my career and was completely focused on my family and my health instead. It's like that moment when a butterfly lands on your finger while you're looking the other way.

I gave a speech a while back, and during the Q&A a student asked me, "What's the biggest failure in your life that has changed you and made you who you are today?"

I'd never really framed it that way before, and as I tried to fashion a response, the answer hit me like a ton of bricks. The biggest failure in my life was my divorce, because it caused so much heartache for so many people I loved. But I've come to realize that the world is never going to collapse if you stumble. In fact, tripping and falling and thrashing now and then are good things, because those mistakes allow us to relate to one another more empathetically. In that vein, cancer has made me much more forgiving and more accepting of shortcomings in myself and in others.

It's also made me more honest. When you say what you think, as long as you say it with compassion, people respond to that authenticity with their own.

With cancer, I've come to realize that all that matters is your most important relationships. I used to chide Andrew because he would take so long getting Wyatt to bed. I'd say, "I got my two kids to bed in ten minutes. You took thirty minutes for your one kid."

But now I'm the one who lingers and cherishes the moment, trying to squeeze as much out of each second of every day, because I just don't know how many I have left. I can sit on the edge of the bed and listen to them talk about whatever's on their mind, or listen to them cry if that's what they need.

I know this is beginning to sound like one of those movies where the corporate big shot gets hit on the head and moves to Vermont (for the record, *Baby Boom* happens to be my favorite movie), but I truly do see beauty in every instant, which I never saw before, and many more opportunities to show and give love. And that same desire to connect with my loved one extends to people at work. I've realized in a profound way that connection is where the goods are.

Driving people to succeed and perform is valuable to a degree. But if that's all you have, you've missed the point. I know it sounds cheesy, but what I've gone through has made me a better wife. I still have a lot of work to do, but I'm more aware of when I'm *not* being a good partner. I'm definitely a better mom. And I'm a better daughter. I'm a better sister and a better friend. I actually *do* the things that I used to only think or dream about. The number of nights I spend with my girlfriends has tripled since I had cancer. I didn't realize how important all of those people were in terms of the fuel that they give me and that I hope I give back to them.

I've always known that being "other directed" is what ultimately makes us happy, but I am more keenly aware of it now. I don't want to fall into the trap of feeling sorry for myself. Focusing on what I can give instead of what I've lost is how I can get through this shit. It counterbalances the awful reality of waiting for that envelope. Will it be good news or bad?

You can't fully understand that gift until you're the one who's been given it, the same way that you can't understand what it's like to wait for that envelope. I'm trying to be a role model for my daughters, but I'm also trying to be a role model for the millions of other women with cancer whose lives aren't as public—or privileged—as mine. Take away the illness, and my life's pretty great, but there are plenty of women who've always had to struggle, and then they get hit with this. I've had so many women say to me, "Go get 'em, Amy!" and I feel an obligation to keep going for them. I try to show that when life really sucks, you can still get up and go to work. Just maybe it's all going to be better; just maybe you're going to live to a ripe old age.

On a flight not long ago, I sat next to the wife of my former boss. We knew each other when we were both younger, and she's now in her fifties. She was complaining about how she looked, how many wrinkles she had, and how her daughter is disgusted by her because, as she put it, "She thinks I'm so old. It's funny, because I look in the mirror and I don't even know who that person is."

Pre-cancer Amy would have commiserated. I would have said, *Oh, I know. Have you done this procedure? Have you tried this cream? I'm thinking about this.*

This time it hit me right in the gut. The first thing I thought was, *God, I hope I have wrinkles. I hope I make it to my fifties. I hope I get to feel a little bit of what you're feeling.*

It seemed self-indulgent to even console her. We're all vain, and I've certainly been distracted by outward appearances. But all of a sudden I wasn't even hearing her, because I was thinking about aging as a blessing in a way I never would have before. I thought, *I'm going to look at my wrinkles in a completely different way, as in, thank God I got one more year's worth. They are my battle scars. They are a source of pride, not something to be ashamed of.*

For all my talk about transformation in place, the truth is I also have a strange recurring daydream that comes to me when I feel overwhelmed or attacked. Andrew and I are living in a cabin in Alaska. There are no cellphones, no media, no New Yorkers, and it makes me happy, because I feel safe. We're hunkering down and focusing only on getting food on the table and creating warmth and shelter. Everyone tells me I wouldn't last three weeks, but someday I'd like to give it a try. In the meantime, I teleport myself there as a little meditation, and it calms me. It makes me smile how much I think about it.

I'm only now beginning to feel physically better. At just past the one-year mark, I'm still weak and tired and often deflated, but strangely I'm getting comfortable enough to make lists again. I'm doing the lint roller; I'm vacuuming; I'm Swiffering. I'm paying attention to whether or not the kids' rooms are clean. I think some part of Andrew really enjoyed the Amy that didn't care. Now he's saying, "Oh, no, the neat freak is back."

For the first anniversary of my mammogram, Robin and I sat down in the same hotel suite where we'd filmed my announcement, and we reflected on life with cancer and what my year had been like.

At one point she asked, "Have you had your day yet?"

"My day?"

"The day where you didn't think about cancer once."

I said, "No."

She smiled her big Robin smile and said, "Well, you're going to have that day. I promise! And when you do, I just want you to lean over to me on the set and say, *I had my day.*"

Acknowledgments

This book was made possible by the phenomenal people I have in my life. First and foremost, I'd like to thank my husband, Andrew, for his loving support and understanding, and for allowing me to write truthfully about the most difficult year of our lives. I have so much love and gratitude for my parents, Joan and Mike Robach, who made me who I am today and love me unconditionally. You gave up an entire eight months of your lives to be by my side, and your love is so powerful and healing.

To my brother, Dr. Eric Robach, who is an intensely private person, thank you for letting me brag about your intelligence, skills, and love, and for being there when I needed you most.

To my little girls, Ava and Annalise, thank you for your smiles, your hugs, and your sweet hearts. You are my strength. To Nate, Aidan, and Wyatt, thank you for your love and your understanding. You are incredibly thoughtful, and it's my privilege and honor to be your stepmom.

I have so many girlfriends to thank—the girls who helped me through those tough chemo months and then helped me celebrate my recovery (and continue to do so every day): Kaitlyn Folmer, Sara

Haines, Jennifer Long, Contessa Brewer, Melissa Lonner, Kristine Johnson, Denise Rehrig, Natasha Singh, Danielle Rossen.

To my loving extended family—my sisters-in-law, Michelle, Lisa, and Jody, and my brothers-in-law, Davis and John; and all of my aunts and uncles, grandparents, and cousins—I can never fully express how much your emails and cards and phone calls have meant to me.

Thank you to my physicians, who continue to monitor my progress and guide me through worries and scares. Dr. Ruth Oratz, Dr. Deborah Axelrod, and Dr. Mihye Choi, you three are truly a dream team.

Thank you to my editor, Jennifer Tung, and all the folks at Ballantine—Gina Centrello, Libby McGuire, Richard Callison, Susan Corcoran, Joe Perez, Toby Ernst, Grant Neumann, Camille Dewing-Val, Benjamin Dreyer, Lisa Feuer, Mark Maguire, Loren Noveck, Pam Alders, and Nina Shield—for your unending support, making my first go at this a pleasurable and incredible experience. Thank you for trusting me to tell my story my way. Thank you to editor Bill Patrick for your help with structure and organization, and for helping me weave my past into my present. Your guidance allowed me to approach and navigate this process confidently.

And to my ABC family. There are so many of you to name! First and foremost, Robin Roberts: Without your guidance and love, none of this would be possible. I owe so much to you, and it is my honor to sit next to you each and every day. You give me strength, hope, and inspiration. To Ben Sherwood, James Goldston, Tom Cibrowski, Michael Corn, and Barbara Fedida, thank you for your unending support and friendship. To my other *GMA* family members, George Stephanopoulos, Lara Spencer, and Ginger Zee, it is a pleasure to work with the best in the business both in front of and behind the camera. To my former ABC colleagues (but my present friends) Sam Champion and Josh Elliott, thank you for bringing a smile to my face and sharing laughter and tears with me when I needed joy and comfort.

To all the women and men who have received a breast cancer diagnosis, to their families and friends who support and love them, and to all those who will one day be diagnosed: This book is for you. Each and every one of you inspires me and gives me the strength to keep fighting. Winning the battle against breast cancer has nothing to do with surviving or dying; it's about spending the time we have on this earth living with gratitude, love, and connection.

About the Author

AMY ROBACH is an American television journalist and anchor for ABC's *Good Morning America*. Previously, she was a national correspondent for NBC News, co-host of the Saturday edition of NBC's *Today*, and an anchor on MSNBC. Over the past twenty years, she has traveled the country and the world interviewing political figures such as Barack Obama, John McCain, Nancy Pelosi, and John Edwards as well as newsmakers like Malala Yousafzai, Oprah Winfrey, and Prince Harry. A Michigan native and graduate of the University of Georgia, Robach lives in New York City with her husband, Andrew Shue, two daughters, and stepsons.

@arobach

Facebook.com/amy.robach.3